Anti-Inflammatory Diet Cookbook For Beginners

2 books in 1 | Simple Meal Plan to Weight Loss and Reduce Inflammation Without Going Crazy | 200 Quick and Easy Recipes to Surprising your Whole Family

By Annette Baker

Copyright © 2021 Annette Baker

All rights reserved.

ISBN: 978-1-80311-082-0 (Paperback)

ISBN: 978-1-80311-083-7 (Hardcover)

Table of Contents

Anti-Inflammatory Diet Cookbook For Men

Chapter 1: Introduction 9

Chapter 2: Breakfast Recipes 10

1) Carrot Rice With Scrambled Eggs 11

2) Egg Muffins With Feta And Quinoa 11

3) Delicious Turmeric Milk 12

4) Green Shakshuka 12

5) Gingered Carrot & Coconut Muffins 13

6) Hot Honey Porridge 13

7) Breakfast Salad.. 13

8) Quick Quinoa With Cinnamon & Chia 14

9) Quinoa And Asparagus Mushroom Frittata... 14

10) Spinach Mushroom Omelet 14

11) Pumpkin & Banana Waffles........................... 15

12) Scrambled Eggs With Smoked Salmon 15

13) Creamy Parmesan Risotto With Mushroom And Cauliflower 15

14) Ranch Roasted Broccoli With Cheddar 16

15) Power Protein Porridge................................. 16

Chapter 3: Lunch & Dinner Recipes 18

16) Smoked Salmon Salad.................................... 19

17) Bean Shawarma Salad.................................... 19

18) Pineapple Fried Rice..................................... 20

19) Lentil Soup 20

20) Delicious Tuna Salad...................................... 21

21) Aioli With Eggs 21

22) Brown Rice And Shitake Miso Soup With Scallions... 21

23) Barbecued Ocean Trout With Garlic And Parsley Dressing 22

24) Buckwheat Noodle Soup................................ 22

25) Easy Salmon Salad....................................... 22

26) Vegetable Soup.. 23

27) Lemony Garlic Shrimp 23

28) Brisket With Blue Cheese.............................. 23

29) Baked Buffalo Cauliflower Chunks 24

30) Garlic Chicken Bake With Basil &tomatoes....24

31) Creamy Turmeric Cauliflower Soup 25

32) Mushroom, Kale, And Sweet Potato Brown Rice 25

33) Baked Tilapia Recipe With Pecan Rosemary Topping 26

34) Black Bean Tortilla Wrap...............................26

35) White Bean Chicken With Winter Green Vegetables 26

36) Herbed Baked Salmon 27

37) Valencia Salad 27

38) "eat Your Greens" Soup.................................27

39) Miso Salmon And Green Beans 28

40) Leek, Chicken, And Spinach Soup 28

41) Dark Choco Bombs 28

42) Italian Stuffed Peppers 29

43) Smoked Trout Wrapped In Lettuce.................29

Chapter 4: Fish & Seafood Recipes 30

44) Broiled Sea Bass 31

45) Spicy Cod 31

46) Smoked Trout Spread 31

47) Tuna And Shallots...32

48) Hot Tuna Steak 32

Chapter 5: Meat Recipes 34

49) Roast Chicken Dal...35

50) Oregano Pork 35

51) Chicken And Avocado Bake 35

52) Five-spice Roasted Duck Breasts 36

53) Pork Chops With Tomato Salsa 36

54) Tuscan Chicken With Tomatoes, Olives, And Zucchini 37

55) Pork Salad 37

56) Lime Pork And Green Beans 37

57) Pork With Chili Zucchinis And Tomatoes........ 38

58) Pork With Olives 38

59) Pork With Nutmeg Squash........................... 38

60) Creamy Pork And Tomatoes 39

61) Lemon Tenderloin 39

62) Chicken With Broccoli 39

63) Pork With Mushrooms And Cucumbers 40

64) Chicken Chopstick 40

65) Balsamic Roast Chicken 40

66) Peach Chicken Treat 41

67) Ground Pork Pan....................................... 41

68) Parsley Pork And Artichokes 41

69) Pork With Thyme Sweet Potatoes 42

70) Curry Pork Mix 42

71) Stir-fried Chicken And Broccoli.................... 42

72) Chicken And Broccoli.................................. 43

73) Pork With Cabbage And Kale 43

74) Mediterranean Chicken Bake With Vegetables 43

75) Hidden Valley Chicken Drummies 44

76) Balsamic Chicken And Beans 44

77) Italian Pork 44

78) Chicken And Brussels Sprouts 45

79) Chicken Divan 45

Chapter 6: Snacks & Desserts Recipes.................... 46

80) Boiled Cabbage.. 47

81) Cereal Mix.. 47

82) Steamed Broccoli 47

83) Berries Cream 47

84) Turmeric Bars 48

85) Cinnamon Apple Mix................................... 48

86) Potato Chips... 48

87) Piquillo Peppers With Cheese 49

88) Lemon Garlic Red Chard 49

89) Rice Pudding... 49

90) Lemony Steamed Asparagus 50

91) Fresh Veggie Bars..................................... 50

92) "cheesy" Brussels Sprouts And Carrots 50

93) Simple Banana Cake 51

94) Massaged Kale Chips.................................. 51

95) Orange And Blackberry Cream.................... 51

96) Lemon Ginger Broccoli And Carrots.............. 51

97) Lemony Cauliflower Rice 52

98) Peppers Avocado Salsa............................... 52

99) Cacao Brownies 52

Chapter 7: Special Recipes 54

100) Caesar Dressing 55

101) Massaged Kale And Crispy Chickpea Salad. 55

102) Garlic Aioli 55

103) Kamut 56

104) Salmon & Beans Salad 56

105) Spinach Salad With Lemony Dressing.......... 56

106) Tender Amaranth Cutlets........................... 57

107) Zoodle Bolognese..................................... 57

108) Stir-fry Sauce.. 58

109) Chicken & Cabbage Salad 58

110) Green Beans With Nuts.............................. 58

111) Green Beans And Mushroom Sauté............. 59

112) Endives And Broccoli................................. 59

113) Beets Stewed With Apples 59

114) Herbed Green Beans 60

115) Peanut Sauce 60

116) Walnut Pesto 60

117) Mushroom And Cauliflower Rice 61

118) Cabbage Slaw With Cashew Dressing......... 61

119) Basic Brown Rice 61

Chapter 8: Anti-Inflammatory Meal Plan for Men 62

Chapter 9: Conclusion... 63

Anti-Inflammatory Diet Cookbook On A Budget

Chapter 1: Introduction 66

Chapter 2: Breakfast Recipes 68

1) Spicy Shakshuka.................................. 69
2) 5-minute Golden Milk 69
3) Breakfast Oatmeal............................... 70
4) No-bake Turmeric Protein Donuts 70
5) Cheddar & Kale Frittata 70
6) Mediterranean Frittata........................... 71
7) Buckwheat Cinnamon And Ginger Granola ... 71
8) Cilantro Pancakes 72
9) Raspberry Grapefruit Smoothie 72
10) Turmeric Oven Scrambled Eggs 72
11) Chia And Oat Breakfast Bran 73
12) Rhubarb, Apple Plus Ginger Muffin Recipe.... 73
13) Breakfast Grains And Fruits 74
14) Perky Paleo Potato & Protein Powder 74
15) Tomato Bruschetta With Basil 74
16) Cinnamon Pancakes With Coconut 75
17) Nutty Blueberry Banana Oatmeal 75
18) Poached Salmon Egg Toast.......................... 76
19) Chia Breakfast Pudding 76
20) Eggs With Cheese 76
21) Tropical Bowls.. 76
22) Shirataki Pasta With Avocado And Cream..... 77
23) Delicious Amaranth Porridge....................... 77
24) Almond Flour Pancakes With Cream Cheese . 77
25) Turkey Apple Breakfast Hash........................ 78
26) Cheesy Flax And Hemp Seeds Muffins 78

Chapter 3: Lunch & Dinner Recipes 80

27) Chicken And Gluten-free Noodle Soup 81
28) Lentil Curry.. 81
29) Chicken And Snap Pea Stir-fry 82
30) Juicy Broccolini With Anchovy Almonds........ 82
31) Shiitake And Spinach Pattie 83
32) Broccoli Cauliflower Salad 83

Chapter 4: Fish & Seafood Recipes 84

33) Broiled White Sea Bass................................ 85
34) Baked Tomato Hake................................. 85
35) Seared Haddock With Beets 85
36) Heartfelt Tuna Melt.................................. 86
37) Lemon Salmon With Kaffir Lime 86

Chapter 5: Meat Recipes 88

38) Peach Chicken Treat 89
39) Ground Pork Pan 89
40) Parsley Pork And Artichokes......................... 89
41) Pork With Thyme Sweet Potatoes 90
42) Curry Pork Mix...................................... 90
43) Stir-fried Chicken And Broccoli 90
44) Chicken And Broccoli 91
45) Pork With Cabbage And Kale 91
46) Mediterranean Chicken Bake With Vegetables 91
47) Hidden Valley Chicken Drummies.................. 92
48) Balsamic Chicken And Beans 92
49) Italian Pork 92
50) Chicken And Brussels Sprouts...................... 93
51) Chicken Divan 93
52) Sumptuous Indian Chicken Curry.................. 93
53) Pork With Balsamic Onion Sauce 94
54) Pork With Pears And Ginger.......................... 94
55) Butter Chicken 94
56) Hot Chicken Wings 95
57) Chicken, Pasta And Snow Peas...................... 95
58) Apricot Chicken Wings............................... 95
59) Champion Chicken Pockets.......................... 96
60) Stovetop Barbecued Chicken Bites 96
61) Chicken And Radish Mix 96
62) Chicken And Sweet Potato Stew.................... 97
63) Rosemary Beef Ribs.................................. 97
64) Chicken, Bell Pepper & Spinach Frittata 98

65) Roast Chicken Dal 98

66) Oregano Pork 98

67) Chicken And Avocado Bake 99

68) Five-spice Roasted Duck Breasts 99

69) Pork Chops With Tomato Salsa 100

70) Tuscan Chicken With Tomatoes, Olives, And Zucchini 100

71) Pork Salad 100

72) Lime Pork And Green Beans 101

73) Pork With Chili Zucchinis And Tomatoes 101

74) Pork With Olives 101

75) Green Enchiladas Chicken Soup 102

Chapter 6: Snacks & Dessert Recipes 104

76) Olives Parsley Spread 105

77) Spinach Cabbage Slaw 105

78) Glazed Pears With Hazelnuts 105

79) Passion Fruit Cream 106

80) Broccoli With Parsley Butter 106

81) Butternut Squash Fries 106

82) Warm Cinnamon-turmeric Almond Milk 107

83) White Fish Ceviche With Avocado 107

84) Mango And Nigella Seeds Stew 107

85) Vanilla Turmeric Orange Juice 108

86) Cauliflower Hummus 108

87) Cinnamon Pecans 108

88) Frozen Blueberry Yogurt Bites 109

Chapter 7: Special Recipes 110

89) Braised Bok Choy With Mushrooms 111

90) White Pizza With Mixed Mushrooms 111

91) Avocado And Herb Spread 111

92) Simple Citrus Vinaigrette Dressing 112

93) Cucumber Salad 112

94) Baked Tomatoes 112

95) Ultimate Roast Potatoes 112

96) Green Beans And Okra 113

97) Herbed Mango Mix 113

98) Devilled Eggs 114

99) Cauliflower Mash 114

100) Chicken Salsa Soup 115

101) Stuffed Pepper Soup 115

102) Honey-lime Vinaigrette With Fresh Herbs 115

103) Rice Pilaf With Almonds 116

104) Rice And Beans 116

105) Parsley Avocado Mix 116

106) Tofu Eggplant Pizza 117

Chapter 8: Anti-Inflammatory Meal Plan On a Budget 118

Chapter 9: Conclusion 119

Anti-Inflammatory Diet Cookbook For Men

A Body Sculpt Meal Plan On a Budget With Quick and Easy Recipes to Weight Loss and Prevent Prostate Cancer | Delicious Meal to Reduce Inflammation

By Annette Baker

Chapter 1: Introduction

There is a myth that men have no special dietary requirements, that they are more resilient and less prone to disease. The reality is that it is not so, men have special requirements in their diet, because of their metabolism, energy consumption and even hormonal changes. Precisely, the anti-inflammatory diet is perfect, because it provides the ideal nutritional contribution for men's needs.

This diet is beneficial for men because inflammation is the common root of numerous chronic pathological processes that men suffer in a higher percentage than women, such as cardiovascular diseases, cancer, Alzheimer's disease or joint inflammation with pain and functional limitation. It also prevents prostate cancer, which according to the American Cancer Society, by 2021 is projected 34,130 deaths due to prostate cancer, you can prevent it with this amazing diet.

What is an anti-inflammatory diet

An anti-inflammatory diet is a dietary regimen whose mission is focused on preventing and/or reducing inflammation in the body. It may be recommended as part of the treatment of a disease, such as an autoimmune disorder, prostate cancer, or simply be part of a healthy diet.

Which foods are allowed in the anti-inflammatory diet

The basis of the anti-inflammatory diet is a higher intake of vegetables, fruits, fish, legumes, poultry, tubers, seeds, whole grains, nuts and olive or coconut oil.

On the other hand, the foods that you should avoid or that are not allowed in the diet are: sodas, processed products, fried foods, sugar, refined flours, alcohol, refined carbohydrates, lard and partially hydrogenated fatty acids or trans fats.

How to start an anti-inflammatory diet

An anti-inflammatory diet is an ancestral diet that has been part of our diet for centuries, therefore it is in our genetic memory and is healthy for everyone. So, starting to follow it will be really easy, and in this cookbook you will find delicious recipes that will allow you to get started in a simple way.

Chapter 2: Breakfast Recipes

1) Carrot Rice With Scrambled Eggs

Preparation Time: **Cooking Time: 3 Hours** **Servings: 3**

Ingredients:

- For Sweet Tamari Soy Sauce
- 3 tbsp tamari sauce (gluten-free)
- 1 tbsp water
- 2-3 tbsp molasses
- For Spicy Mix-ins
- 3 garlic cloves
- 1 small shallot (sliced)
- 2 long red chilies
- Pinch of ground ginger
- For the Carrot Rice:
- 2 Tbsp sesame oil

- 5 eggs
- 4 large carrots
- 8 ounces sausage (chicken or any type of – gluten-free and minced).
- 1 tbsp sweet soy sauce
- 1 cup bean sprouts
- 1/2 cup fined diced broccoli
- salt and pepper to taste
- For Garnish:
- Cilantro
- Asian chili sauce
- Sesame seeds

Directions:

⇒ For the Sauce:

⇒ In a saucepan, boil molasses, water, and tamari at a high flame.

⇒ Lower the flame after the sauce boils and cook till molasses is completely dissolved.

⇒ Place the sauce in a separate bowl.

⇒ For the Carrot Rice:

⇒ In a bowl, combine ginger, garlic, onion, and red chilies.

⇒ To make rice out of the carrots, spiralize the carrots in a spiralizer.

⇒ Pulse the spiralized carrots in a food processor.

⇒ Cut broccoli into small dice like pieces

⇒ Add the sausage, carrots, broccoli, and the bean sprouts into the bowl of onion, ginger, garlic, and chilies.

⇒ Add the spicy mix of vegetables and the tamari sauce in the slow cooker pot.

⇒ Set the cooker on high heat for 3 hours or low heat for 6 hours.

⇒ Scramble two eggs in a non-stick frying pan or skillet.

⇒ Dish out the carrot rice and add scrambled eggs on top.

⇒ Garnish with sesame seeds, Asian chili sauce, and cilantro.

Nutrition: Calories 230 mg Total Fat: 13.7g Carbohydrates: 15.9g Protein: 12.2g Sugar: 8g Fiber 4.4g Sodium: 1060 mg Cholesterol: 239mg.

2) Egg Muffins With Feta And Quinoa

Preparation Time: **Cooking Time: 30 Minutes** **Servings: 12**

Ingredients:

- Eggs, eight
- Tomatoes, chopped, one cup
- Salt, one quarter teaspoon
- Feta cheese, one cup
- Quinoa, one cup cooked

- Olive oil, two teaspoons
- Oregano, fresh chop, one tablespoon
- Black olives, chopped, one quarter cup
- Onion, chopped, one quarter cup
- Baby spinach, chopped, two cups

Directions:

⇒ Heat oven to 350. Spray oil a muffin pan with twelve cups. Cook spinach, oregano, olives, onion, and tomatoes for five minutes in the olive oil over medium heat. Beat eggs. Add the cooked mix of veggies to the eggs with the cheese and salt. Spoon mixture into muffin cups.

⇒ Bake thirty minutes. These will remain fresh in the fridge for two days. To eat, just wrap in a paper towel and warm in the microwave for thirty seconds.

Nutrition: Calorie 113 carbs 5 gramsprotein 6 gramsfat 7 gramssugar 1-gram

3) Delicious Turmeric Milk

Preparation Time: **Cooking Time: 5 Minutes**   **Servings:2**

Ingredients:

- 1½ cups coconut milk, unsweetened
- 1½ cups almond milk, unsweetened
- ¼ teaspoon ground ginger
- 1½ teaspoon ground turmeric
- 1 tablespoon coconut oil
- ¼ teaspoon ground cinnamon

Directions:

⇒ Put the coconut and almond milk in a small pot and heat over medium heat, add the ginger, oil, turmeric and cinnamon.

⇒ Mix and cook for 5 minutes, divide into bowls and serve.

⇒ Enjoy!

Nutrition: calories 171, fat 3, fiber 4, carbs 6, protein 7

4) Green Shakshuka

Preparation Time: **Cooking Time: 25 Minutes**   **Servings:4**

Ingredients:

- 2 tablespoons extra-virgin olive oil
- 1 onion, minced
- 2 garlic cloves, minced
- 1 jalapeño, seeded and minced
- 1-pound spinach (thawed if frozen)
- 1 teaspoon dried cumin
- ¾ teaspoon coriander
- Salt and freshly ground black pepper
- 2 tablespoons harissa
- ½ cup vegetable broth
- 8 large eggs
- Chopped fresh parsley, as needed for serving
- Chopped fresh cilantro, as needed for serving
- Red-pepper flakes, as needed for serving

Directions:

⇒ Preheat the oven to 350 ° F.

⇒ Heat the olive oil inside a large, oven-safe skillet, over medium heat. Add the onion and sauté for 4 to 5 minutes. Stir in the garlic and jalapeño, then sauté 1 minute more until fragrant.

⇒ Add the spinach and cook until fully wilted if fresh, 4 to 5 minutes or 1 to 2 minutes if thawed from frozen, until heated through.

⇒ Season with cumin, pepper, coriander, salt, and harissa. Cook for approximately 1 minute, until fragrant.

⇒ Switch the mixture to a food processor bowl or a blender and puree until it is coarse. Connect the broth and purée until smooth and thick.

⇒ Wipe the skillet out and dust it with nonstick cooking spray. Pour the spinach mixture into the pan back and make eight circular wells using a wooden spoon.

⇒ Crack the eggs in the pipes, softly. Switch the skillet to the oven and cook for 20 to 25 minutes until the egg whites are set fully, but the yolks are still a little jiggly.

⇒ Sprinkle with parsley, cilantro, and red pepper flakes on the shakshuka, to taste. Serve straight away.

Nutrition: 251 calories17g fat10g carbs17g protein3g sugars

5) Gingered Carrot & Coconut Muffins

Preparation Time: **Cooking Time: 20-22 Minutes**   **Servings: 12**

Ingredients:

- 2 cups blanched almond flour
- ½ cup unsweetened coconut shreds
- 1 tsp baking soda
- ½ teaspoon allspice
- ½ teaspoon ground ginger
- Pinch of ground cloves
- Salt, to taste

- 3 organic eggs
- ½ cup organic honey
- ½ cup coconut oil
- 1 cup carrot, peeled and grated
- 2 tablespoons fresh ginger, peeled and grated
- ¾ cup raisins, soaked in water for 15 minutes and drained

Directions:

⇒ Preheat the oven to 350 degrees F. Grease 12 cups of a large muffin tin.

⇒ In a sizable bowl, mix together flour, coconut shreds, baking soda, spices and salt.

⇒ In another bowl, add eggs, honey, and oil and beat till well combined.

⇒ Add egg mixture into flour mixture and mix till well combined.

⇒ Fold in carrot, ginger and raisins.

⇒ Place the mix into prepared muffin cups evenly.

⇒ Bake approximately 20-22 minutes or till a toothpick inserted inside center arrives clean.

Nutrition: Calories: 352, Fat: 13g, Carbohydrates: 33g, Fiber: 9g, Protein: 15g

6) Hot Honey Porridge

Preparation Time: **Cooking Time:**   **Servings: 4**

Ingredients:

- ¼ c. honey
- ½ c. rolled oats

- 3 c. boiling water
- ¾ c. bulgur wheat

Directions:

⇒ Place the bulgur wheat and rolled oats into a saucepan. Add the boiling water and stir to combine.

⇒ Place pan over high heat and bring to a boil. Once boiling, reduce heat to low, then cover and simmer for 10 minutes, stirring occasionally.

⇒ Remove from heat, stir in honey, and serve immediately.

Nutrition: Calories: 172, Fat:1 g, Carbs:40 g, Protein:4 g, Sugars:5 g, Sodium:20 mg

7) Breakfast Salad

Preparation Time: **Cooking Time: 0 Minutes**   **Servings: 4**

Ingredients:

- 27 ounces kale salad mixed with dried fruit
- 1 ½ cups blueberries
- 15 ounces beets, cooked, peeled and cubed
- ¼ cup olive oil
- 2 tablespoons apple cider vinegar

- 1 teaspoon turmeric powder
- 1 tablespoon lemon juice
- 1 garlic clove, minced
- 1 teaspoon fresh grated ginger
- A pinch of black pepper

Directions:

⇒ In a salad bowl, mix the kale and dried fruit with beets and blueberries. In a separate bowl, mix the oil with the vinegar, turmeric, lemon juice, garlic, ginger and a pinch of black pepper, whisk well then pour over the salad, toss and serve.

⇒ Enjoy!

Nutrition: calories 188, fat 4, fiber 6, carbs 14, protein 7

8) Quick Quinoa With Cinnamon & Chia

Preparation Time: **Cooking Time: 3 Minutes**   **Servings:2**

Ingredients:

- 2-cups quinoa, pre-cooked
- 1-cup cashew milk
- ½-tsp ground cinnamon
- 1-cup fresh blueberries
- ¼-cup walnuts, toasted
- 2-tsp raw honey
- 1-Tbsp chia seeds

Directions:

⇒ Over medium-low heat, add the quinoa and cashew milk in a saucepan. Stir in the cinnamon, blueberries, and walnuts. Cook slowly for three minutes.

⇒ Remove the pan from the heat. Stir in the honey. Garnish with chia seeds on top before serving.

Nutrition: Calories 887Fat: 29.5gProtein: 44. Sodium: 85mgTotal Carbs: 129.3gDietary Fiber: 18.5g

9) Quinoa And Asparagus Mushroom Frittata

Preparation Time: **Cooking Time: 30 Minutes**   **Servings:3**

Ingredients:

- 2 tablespoons olive oil
- 1 cup sliced mushrooms
- 1 cup asparagus, cut into 1-inch pieces
- ½ cup chopped tomato
- 6 large eggs, pasture-raised
- 2 large egg whites, pasture-raised
- ¼ cup non-dairy milk
- 1 cup quinoa, cooked according to the package
- 3 tablespoons chopped basil
- 1 tablespoon chopped parsley, garnish
- Salt and pepper to taste

Directions:

⇒ Preheat the oven to 3500F.

⇒ In a skillet, heat the olive oil over medium flame.

⇒ Stir in the mushrooms and asparagus.

⇒ Season with salt and pepper to taste. Sauté for 7 minutes or until the mushrooms and asparagus have browned.

⇒ Add the tomatoes and cook for another 3 minutes. Set aside.

⇒ Meanwhile, mix the eggs, egg white, and milk in a mixing bowl. Set aside.

⇒ Place in a baking dish the quinoa and top with the vegetable mixture. Pour in the egg mixture.

⇒ Place in the oven and bake for 20 minutes or until the eggs have set.

Nutrition: Calories 450Total Fat 37gSaturated Fat 5gTotal Carbs 17gNet Carbs 14gProtein 12gSugar: 2gFiber: 3gSodium: 60mgPotassium 349mg

10) Spinach Mushroom Omelet

Preparation Time: **Cooking Time: 15 Minutes**   **Servings:2**

Ingredients:

- Olive oil, one tablespoon + one tablespoon
- Spinach, fresh, chopped, one- and one-half cup
- Green onion, one diced
- Eggs, three
- Feta cheese, one ounce
- Mushrooms, button, five sliced
- Red onion, diced, one quarter cup

Directions:

⇒ Sauté the mushrooms, onions, and spinach for three minutes in one tablespoon of olive oil and set to the side. Beat the eggs well and cook them in the other tablespoon of olive oil for three to four minutes until edges begin to brown.

⇒ Sprinkle all the other ingredients onto half of the omelet and fold the other half over the sautéed ingredients. Cook for one minute on each side.

Nutrition: Calories 337 fat 25 grams protein 22 grams carbs 5.4 grams sugar 1.3 grams fiber 1-gram

11) Pumpkin & Banana Waffles

Preparation Time: **Cooking Time: 5 Minutes**   **Servings:4**

Ingredients:

- ½ cup almond flour
- ½ cup coconut flour
- 1 tsp baking soda
- 1½ teaspoons ground cinnamon
- ¾ teaspoon ground ginger
- ½ teaspoon ground cloves
- ½ teaspoon ground nutmeg

- Salt, to taste
- 2 tablespoons olive oil
- 5 large organic eggs
- ¾ cup almond milk
- ½ cup pumpkin puree
- 2 medium bananas, peeled and sliced

Directions:

⇒ Preheat the waffle iron and after that grease it.

⇒ In a sizable bowl, mix together flours, baking soda and spices.

⇒ In a blender, add remaining ingredients and pulse till smooth.

⇒ Add flour mixture and pulse till

⇒ In preheated waffle iron, add required quantity of mixture.

⇒ Cook approximately 4-5 minutes.

⇒ Repeat using the remaining mixture.

Nutrition: Calories: 357.2, Fat: 28.5g, Carbohydrates: 19.7g, Fiber: 4g, Protein: 14g

12) Scrambled Eggs With Smoked Salmon

Preparation Time: **Cooking Time: 10 Minutes**   **Servings:2**

Ingredients:

- 4 eggs
- 2 tablespoons coconut milk
- Fresh chives, chopped

- 4 slices of wild-caught smoked salmon, chopped
- Salt to taste

Directions:

⇒ In a bowl, whisk the egg, coconut milk, and chives.

⇒ Grease the skillet with oil and heat over medium-low heat.

⇒ Pour the egg mixture and scramble the eggs while cooking.

⇒ When the eggs start to settle, add in the smoked salmon and cook for 2 more minutes.

Nutrition: Calories 349Total Fat 23gSaturated Fat 4gTotal Carbs 3gNet Carbs 1gProtein 29gSugar: 2gFiber: 2gSodium: 466mgPotassium 536mg

13) Creamy Parmesan Risotto With Mushroom And Cauliflower

Preparation Time: **Cooking Time: 18 Minutes**   **Servings:2**

Ingredients:

- 1 clove of garlic, peeled, sliced
- ½ cup heavy cream
- ½ cup cauliflower, riced

- ½ cup mushrooms, sliced
- Coconut oil, for frying
- Parmesan cheese, grated, for topping

Directions:

⇒ Take a skillet pan, place it over medium-high heat, add coconut oil and when it melts, add garlic and mushrooms and cook for 4 minutes or until sauté.

⇒ Then add cauliflower and cream into the pan, stir well and simmer for 12 minutes.

⇒ Transfer the risotto to a plate, top with cheese and then serve.

Nutrition: Calories 179, Total Fat 17.8g, Total Carbs 4.4g, Protein 2.8g, Sugar 2.1g, Sodium 61mg

14) Ranch Roasted Broccoli With Cheddar

Preparation Time:	**Cooking Time: 30 Minutes**	**Servings:2**

Ingredients:

- 1½ cups broccoli florets
- Salt and freshly cracked black pepper, to taste
- 1/8 cup ranch dressing

- 1/8 cup heavy whipping cream
- ¼ cup shredded sharp cheddar cheese
- 1 tbsp olive oil

Directions:

⇒ Switch on the oven, then set its temperature to 375°F and let it preheat.

⇒ Meanwhile, take a medium bowl, add florets in it along with remaining ingredients and stir until well combined.

⇒ Take a casserole dish, grease it with oil, spoon in prepared mixture and bake for 30 minutes until thoroughly cooked.

⇒ When done, let casserole cool for 5 minutes and then serve.

Nutrition: Calories 111, Total Fat 7.7g, Total Carbs 5.7g, Protein 5.8g, Sugar 1.6g, Sodium 198mg

15) Power Protein Porridge

Preparation Time:	**Cooking Time: 8 Minutes**	**Servings:2**

Ingredients:

- ¼-cup walnut or pecan halves, roughly chopped
- ¼-cup toasted coconut, unsweetened
- 2-Tbsps hemp seeds
- 2-Tbsps whole chia seeds
- ¾-cup almond milk, unsweetened
- ¼-cup coconut milk

- ¼-cup almond butter, roasted
- ½-tsp turmeric, ground
- 1-Tbsp extra virgin coconut oil or MCT oil
- 2-Tbsps erythritol or 5-10 drops liquid stevia (optional)
- A pinch of ground black pepper
- ½-tsp cinnamon or ½-tsp vanilla powder

Directions:

⇒ Put the walnuts, flaked coconut, and hemp seeds in a hot saucepan. Roast the mixture for 2 minutes, or until fragrant. Stir a few times to prevent burning. Transfer the roasted mix in a bowl. Set aside.

⇒ Combine the almond and coco milk in a small saucepan placed over medium heat. Heat the mixture.

⇒ After heating, but not boiling, switch off the heat. Add all the remaining ingredients. Mix well until thoroughly combined. Set aside for 10 minutes.

⇒ Combine half of the roasted mix with the porridge. Scoop the porridge into two serving bowls. Sprinkle each bowl with the remaining half of the roasted mixture and cinnamon powder. Serve the porridge immediately.

Nutrition: Calories 572Fat: 19gProtein: 28.6gSodium: 87mgTotal Carbs: 81.5gDietary Fiber: 10g

Chapter 3: Lunch & Dinner Recipes

16) Smoked Salmon Salad

Ingredients:

- 2 baby fennel bulbs, thinly sliced, some fronds reserved
- 1 tablespoon salted baby capers, rinsed, drained
- ½ cup natural yogurt
- 2 tablespoons parsley, chopped
- 1 tablespoon lemon juice, freshly squeezed
- 2 tablespoons fresh chives, chopped
- 1 tablespoon chopped fresh tarragon

- 180g sliced smoked salmon, low-salt
- ½ red onion, sliced thinly
- 1 teaspoon lemon rind, finely grated
- ½ cup French green lentils, rinsed
- 60g fresh baby spinach
- ½ avocado, sliced
- A pinch of caster sugar

Directions:

⇒ Put water in a large saucepan with water and boil over moderate heat. Once boiling; cook the lentils until tender, for 20 minutes; drain well.

⇒ In the meantime, heat a chargrill pan over high heat in advance. Spray the fennel slices with some oil & cook until tender, for 2 minutes per side.

⇒ Process the chives, parsley, yogurt, tarragon, lemon rind, and capers in a food processor until completely smooth and then season with pepper to taste.

⇒ Place the onion with sugar, juice & a pinch of salt in a large-sized mixing bowl. Set aside for a couple of minutes and then drain.

⇒ Combine the lentils with onion, fennel, avocado, and spinach in a large-sized mixing bowl. Evenly divide among the plates and then top with the fish. Sprinkle with the leftover fennel fronds & more of fresh parsley. Drizzle with the green goddess dressing. Enjoy.

Nutrition: kcal 368 Fat: 14 g Fiber: 8 g Protein: 20 g

17) Bean Shawarma Salad

Ingredients:

- For Preparing Salad
- 20 Pita chips
- 5-ounces Spring lettuce
- 10 Cherry tomatoes
- ¾ Cup fresh parsley
- ¼ Cup red onion (chop)
- For Chickpeas
- 1tbsp Olive oil
- 1 Heading-tbsp cumin and turmeric
- ½ Heading-tbsp paprika and coriander powder

- 1 Pinch black pepper
- ½ Scant Kosher salt
- ¼tbsp Ginger and cinnamon powder
- For Preparing Dressing
- 3 Garlic Cloves
- 1tbsp Dried drill
- 1tbsp Lime juice
- Water
- ½ Cup hummus

Directions:

⇒ Place a rack in the already preheated oven (204C). Mix chickpeas with all spices and herbs.

⇒ Place a thin layer of chickpeas on the baking sheet and bake it almost for 20 minutes. Bake it until the beans are golden brown.

⇒ For preparing the dressing, mix all ingredients in a whisking bowl and blend it. Add water gradually for appropriate smoothness.

⇒ Mix all herbs and spices for preparing salad.

⇒ For serving, add pita chips and beans in the salad and drizzle some dressing over it.

Nutrition: Calories 173Carbs: 8gFat: 6gProtein: 19g

18) Pineapple Fried Rice

Preparation Time: **Cooking Time: 20 Minutes** **Servings: 4**

Ingredients:

- 2 carrots, peeled and grated
- 2 green onions, sliced
- 3 tablespoons soy sauce
- 1/2 cup ham, diced
- 1 tablespoon sesame oil
- 2 cups canned/fresh pineapple, diced
- 1/2 teaspoon ginger powder
- 3 cups brown rice, cooked

- 1/4 teaspoon white pepper
- 2 tablespoons olive oil
- 1/2 cup frozen peas
- 2 garlic cloves, minced
- 1/2 cup frozen corn
- 1 onion, diced

Directions:

⇒ Put 1 tablespoon sesame oil, 3 tablespoons soy sauce, 2 pinches of white pepper, and 1/2 teaspoon ginger powder in a bowl. Mix well and keep it aside.

⇒ Preheat oil in a skillet. Add the garlic along with the diced onion. Cook for about 3-4 minutes, stirring often.

⇒ Add 1/2 cup frozen peas, grated carrots, and 1/2 cup frozen corn. Stir until veggies are tender, just for few minutes.

⇒ Stir in soy sauce mixture, 2 cups of diced pineapple, ½ cup chopped ham, 3 cups cooked brown rice, and sliced green onions. Cook for about 2-3 minutes, stirring often. Serve!

Nutrition: 252 calories 12.8 g fat 33 g total carbs 3 g protein

19) Lentil Soup

Preparation Time: **Cooking Time: 30 Minutes** **Servings: 2**

Ingredients:

- 2 Carrots, medium & diced
- 2 tbsp. Lemon Juice, fresh
- 1 tbsp. Turmeric Powder
- 1/3 cup Lentils, cooked
- 1 tbsp. Almonds, chopped
- 1 Celery Stalk, diced
- 1 bunch of Parsley, chopped freshly
- 1 Yellow Onion, large & chopped

- Black Pepper, freshly grounded
- 1 Parsnip, medium & chopped
- ½ tsp. Cumin Powder
- 3 ½ cups Water
- ½ tsp. Pink Himalayan Salt
- 4 kale leaves, chopped roughly

Directions:

⇒ To start with, place carrots, parsnip, one tablespoon of water and onion in a medium-sized pot over medium heat.

⇒ Cook the vegetable mixture for 5 minutes while stirring it occasionally.

⇒ Next, stir in the lentils and spices into it. Combine well.

⇒ After that, pour water to the pot and bring the mixture to a boil.

⇒ Now, reduce the heat to low and allow it to simmer for 20 minutes.

⇒ Off the heat and remove it from the stove. Add the kale, lemon juice, parsley, and salt to it.

⇒ Then, give a good stir until everything comes together.

⇒ Top it with almonds and serve it hot.

Nutrition: Calories: 242KcalProteins: 10gCarbohydrates: 46gFat: 4g

20) Delicious Tuna Salad

Preparation Time: **Cooking Time: 15 Minutes**   **Servings:2**

Ingredients:

- 2 cans tuna packed in water (5oz each), drained
- ¼ cup mayonnaise
- 2 tablespoons fresh basil, chopped
- 1 tablespoon lemon juice, freshly squeezed
- 2 tablespoons fire-roasted red peppers, chopped
- ¼ cup kalamata or mixed olives, chopped
- 2 large vine-ripened tomatoes
- 1 tablespoon capers
- 2 tablespoons red onion, minced
- Pepper & salt to taste

Directions:

⇒ Add all the items (except tomatoes) together in a large-sized mixing bowl; give the ingredients a good stir until combined well. Slice the tomatoes into sixths and then gently pry it open.

⇒ Scoop the prepared tuna salad mixture into the middle; serve immediately & enjoy.

Nutrition: kcal 405 Fat: 24 g Fiber: 3.2 g Protein: 37 g

21) Aioli With Eggs

Preparation Time: **Cooking Time: 0 Minutes**   **Servings:12**

Ingredients:

- 2 egg yolks
- 1 garlic, grated
- 2 Tbsp. water
- ½ cup extra virgin olive oil
- ¼ cup lemon juice, fresh squeezed, pips removed
- ¼ tsp. sea salt
- Dash of cayenne pepper powder
- Pinch of white pepper, to taste

Directions:

⇒ Pour garlic, egg yolks, salt, and water into blender; process until smooth. Put in olive oil in a slow stream until dressing emulsifies.

⇒ Add in remaining ingredients. Taste; adjust seasoning if needed. Pour into an airtight container; use as needed.

Nutrition: Calories 100Carbs: 1gFat: 11gProtein: 0g

22) Brown Rice And Shitake Miso Soup With Scallions

Preparation Time: **Cooking Time: 45 Minutes**   **Servings:4**

Ingredients:

- 2 tablespoons sesame oil
- 1 cup thinly sliced shiitake mushroom caps
- 1 garlic clove, minced
- 1 (1½-inch) piece fresh ginger, peeled and sliced
- 1 cup medium-grain brown rice
- ½ teaspoon salt
- 1 tablespoon white miso
- 2 scallions, thinly sliced
- 2 tablespoons finely chopped fresh cilantro

Directions:

⇒ Heat-up the oil over medium-high heat in a large pot.

⇒ Add the mushrooms, garlic, and ginger and sauté until the mushrooms begin to soften about 5 minutes.

⇒ Put the rice and stir to coat with the oil evenly. Add 2 cups of water and salt and boil.

⇒ Simmer within 30 to 40 minutes. Use a little of the soup broth to soften the miso, then stir it into the pot until well blended.

⇒ Mix in the scallions plus cilantro, then serve.

Nutrition: Calories 265 Total Fat: 8g Total Carbohydrates: 43g Sugar: 2g Fiber: 3gProtein: 5gSodium: 456mg

23) Barbecued Ocean Trout With Garlic And Parsley Dressing

Preparation Time: **Cooking Time: 25 Minutes** **Servings: 8**

Ingredients:

- 3 ½ pounds piece of trout fillet, preferably ocean trout, boned, skin on
- 4 cloves of garlic, sliced thinly
- 2 tablespoons capers, coarsely chopped
- ½ cup flat-leaf parsley leaves, fresh
- 1 red chili, preferably long; sliced thinly
- 2 tablespoons lemon juice, freshly squeezed
- ½ cup olive oil
- Lemon wedges, to serve

Directions:

⇒ Brush the trout with approximately 2 tablespoons of oil; ensure that all sides are coated nicely. Preheat your barbecue over high heat, preferably with a closed hood. Decrease the heat to medium; place the coated trout on the barbecue plate, preferably on the skin-side. Cook until partially cooked and turn golden, for a couple of minutes. Carefully turn the trout; cook until cooked through, for 12 to 15 minutes, with the hood closed. Transfer the fillet to a large-sized serving platter.

⇒ In the meantime, heat the leftover oil; garlic over low heat in a small-sized saucepan until just heated through; garlic begins to change its color. Remove, then stir in the capers, lemon juice, chili. Drizzle the trout with the prepared dressing and then sprinkle with the fresh parsley leaves. Immediately serve with fresh lemon wedges, enjoy.

Nutrition: kcal 170 Fat: 30 g Fiber: 2 g Protein: 37 g

24) Buckwheat Noodle Soup

Preparation Time: **Cooking Time: 25 Minutes** **Servings: 4**

Ingredients:

- 2 cups Bok Choy, chopped
- 3 tbsp. Tamari
- 3 bundles of Buckwheat Noodles
- 2 cups Edamame Beans
- 7 oz. Shiitake Mushrooms, chopped
- 4 cups Water
- 1 tsp. Ginger, grated
- Dash of Salt
- 1 Garlic Clove, grated

Directions:

⇒ First, place water, ginger, soy sauce, and garlic in a medium-sized pot over medium heat.

⇒ Bring the ginger-soy sauce mixture to a boil and then stir in the edamame and shiitake to it.

⇒ Continue cooking for further 7 minutes or until tender.

⇒ Next, cook the soba noodles by following the Directions: given in the packet until cooked. Wash and drain well.

⇒ Now, add the bok choy to shiitake mixture and cook for further one minute or until the bok choy is wilted.

⇒ Finally, divide the soba noodles among the serving bowls and top it with the mushroom mixture.

Nutrition: Calories: 234Kcal Proteins: 14.2g Carbohydrates: 35.1g Fat: 4g

25) Easy Salmon Salad

Preparation Time: **Cooking Time: 0 Minutes** **Servings: 1**

Ingredients:

- 1 cup of organic arugula
- 1 can of wild-caught salmon
- ½ of an avocado, sliced
- 1 tablespoon of olive oil
- 1 teaspoon of Dijon mustard
- 1 teaspoon of sea salt

Directions:

⇒ Start by whisking the olive oil, Dijon mustard, and sea salt together in a mixing bowl to make the dressing. Set aside.

⇒ Assemble the salad with the arugula as the base, and top with the salmon and sliced avocado.

⇒ Drizzle with the dressing.

Nutrition: Total Carbohydrates 7g Dietary Fiber: 5g Protein: 48g Total Fat: 37g Calories: 553

26) Vegetable Soup

Preparation Time:	Cooking Time: 40 Minutes	Servings:4

Ingredients:

- 1 tbsp. Coconut Oil
- 2 cups Kale, chopped
- 2 Celery Stalks, diced
- ½ of 15 oz. can of White Beans, drained & rinsed
- 1 Onion, large & diced
- ¼ tsp. Black Pepper
- 1 Carrot, medium & diced
- 2 cups Cauliflower, cut into florets
- 1 tsp. Turmeric, grounded
- 1 tsp. Sea Salt
- 3 Garlic cloves, minced
- 6 cups Vegetable Broth

Directions:

⇒ To start with, heat oil in a large pot over medium-low heat.

⇒ Stir in the onion to the pot and sauté it for 5 minutes or until softened.

⇒ Put the carrot plus celery to the pot and continue cooking for another 4 minutes or until the veggies softened.

⇒ Now, spoon in the turmeric, garlic, and ginger to the mixture. Stir well.

⇒ Cook the veggie mixture for 1 minute or until fragrant.

⇒ Then, pour the vegetable broth along with salt and pepper and bring the mixture to a boil.

⇒ Once it starts boiling, add the cauliflower. Reduce the heat and simmer the vegetable mixture for 13 to 15 minutes or until the cauliflower is softened.

⇒ Finally, add the beans and kale—Cook within 2 minutes.

⇒ Serve it hot.

Nutrition: Calories 192KcalProteins:12.6gCarbohydrates: 24.6gFat: 6.4g

27) Lemony Garlic Shrimp

Preparation Time:	Cooking Time: 15 Minutes	Servings:4

Ingredients:

- 1 and ¼ pounds shrimp, boiled or steamed
- 3 tablespoons garlic, minced
- ¼ cup lemon juice
- 2 tablespoons olive oil
- ¼ cup parsley

Directions:

⇒ Take a small skillet and place it over medium heat, add garlic and oil and stir cook for 1 minute.

⇒ Add parsley, lemon juice and season with salt and pepper accordingly.

⇒ Add shrimp in a large bowl and transfer the mixture from the skillet over the shrimp.

⇒ Chill and serve.

Nutrition: Calories: 130Fat: 3gCarbohydrates: 2gProtein: 22g

28) Brisket With Blue Cheese

Preparation Time:	Cooking Time: 8 Hrs. 10 Minutes	Servings:6

Ingredients:

- 1 cup of water
- 1/2 tbsp garlic paste
- 1/4 cup soy sauce
- 1 ½ lb. corned beef brisket
- 1/3 teaspoon ground coriander
- 1/4 teaspoon cloves, ground
- 1 tbsp olive oil
- 1 shallot, chopped
- 2 oz. blue cheese, crumbled
- Cooking spray

Directions:

⇒ Place a pan over moderate heat and add oil to heat.

⇒ Toss in shallots and stir and cook for 5 minutes.

⇒ Stir in garlic paste and cook for 1 minute.

⇒ Transfer it to the slow cooker, greased with cooking spray.

⇒ Place brisket in the same pan and sear until golden from both sides.

⇒ Transfer the beef to the slow cooker along with other ingredients except for cheese.

⇒ Put on its lid and cook for 8 hrs. on low heat.

⇒ Garnish with cheese and serve.

Nutrition: Calories 397, Protein 23.5g, Fat 31.4g, Carbs 3.9g, Fiber 0 g

29) Baked Buffalo Cauliflower Chunks

Preparation Time: **Cooking Time: 35 Minutes**   **Servings:2**

Ingredients:

- ¼-cup water
- ¼-cup banana flour
- A pinch of salt and pepper
- 1-pc medium cauliflower, cut into bite-size pieces

- ½-cup hot sauce
- 2-Tbsp.s butter, melted
- Blue cheese or ranch dressing (optional)

Directions:

⇒ Preheat your oven to 425°F. Meanwhile, line a baking pan with foil.

⇒ Combine the water, flour, and a pinch of salt and pepper in a large mixing bowl.

⇒ Mix well until thoroughly combined.

⇒ Add the cauliflower; toss to coat thoroughly.

⇒ Transfer the mixture to the baking pan. Bake for 15 minutes, flipping once.

⇒ While baking, combine the hot sauce and butter in a small bowl.

⇒ Pour the sauce over the baked cauliflower.

⇒ Return the baked cauliflower to the oven, and bake further for 20 minutes.

⇒ Serve immediately with a ranch dressing on the side, if desired.

Nutrition: Calories: 168Cal Fat: 5.6gProtein: 8.4gCarbs: 23.8gFiber: 2.8g

30) Garlic Chicken Bake With Basil &tomatoes

Preparation Time: **Cooking Time: 30 Minutes**   **Servings:4**

Ingredients:

- ½ medium yellow onion
- 2tbsp Olive oil
- 3 Minced Garlic Cloves
- 1 Cup Basil (loosely cut)
- 1.lb Boneless chicken breast

- 14.5-ounces Italian chop tomatoes
- Salt & pepper
- 4 Medium zucchinis (spiralized into noodles)
- 1tbsp crushed red pepper
- 2tbsp Olive oil

Directions:

⇒ Pound the chicken pieces with a pan for fast cooking. Sprinkle salt, pepper, and oil on chicken pieces and marinate both sides of chicken equally.

⇒ Fry chicken pieces on a large hot skillet for 2-3 minutes on each side.

⇒ Sautee onion in the same skillet pan until it's brown. Add tomatoes, basil leaves, and garlic in it.

⇒ Simmer it for 3 minutes and add all spices and chicken in the skillet.

⇒ Serve it on the plate along with saucy zoodles.

Nutrition: Calories 44Carbs: 7gFat: 0gProtein: 2g

31) Creamy Turmeric Cauliflower Soup

Preparation Time: **Cooking Time: 15 Minutes**   **Servings:4**

Ingredients:

- 2 tablespoons extra-virgin olive oil
- 1 leek, white part only, thinly sliced
- 3 cups cauliflower florets
- 1 garlic clove, peeled
- 1 (1¼-inch) piece fresh ginger, peeled and sliced
- 1½ teaspoons turmeric

- ½ teaspoon salt
- ¼ teaspoon freshly ground black pepper
- ¼ teaspoon ground cumin
- 3 cups vegetable broth
- 1 cup full-Fat: coconut milk
- ¼ cup finely chopped fresh cilantro

Directions:

⇒ Heat-up the oil over high heat in a large pot.

⇒ Sauté the leek within 3 to 4 minutes.

⇒ Put the cauliflower, garlic, ginger, turmeric, salt, pepper, and cumin and sauté for 1 to 2 minutes.

⇒ Put the broth, and boil.

⇒ Simmer within 5 minutes.

⇒ Purée the soup using an immersion blender until smooth.

⇒ Stir in the coconut milk and cilantro, heat through, and serve.

Nutrition: Calories 264 Total Fat: 23g Total Carbohydrates: 12g Sugar: 5g Fiber: 4gProtein: 7gSodium: 900mg

32) Mushroom, Kale, And Sweet Potato Brown Rice

Preparation Time: **Cooking Time: 50 Minutes**   **Servings:4**

Ingredients:

- ¼ cup extra-virgin olive oil
- 4 cups coarsely chopped kale leaves
- 2 leeks, white parts only, thinly sliced
- 1 cup sliced mushrooms
- 2 garlic cloves, minced
- 2 cups peeled sweet potatoes cut into ½-inch dice

- 1 cup of brown rice
- 2 cups vegetable broth
- 1 teaspoon salt
- ¼ teaspoon freshly ground black pepper
- ¼ cup freshly squeezed lemon juice
- 2 tablespoons finely chopped fresh flat-leaf parsley

Directions:

⇒ Heat the oil over high heat.

⇒ Add the kale, leeks, mushrooms, and garlic and sauté until soft, about 5 minutes.

⇒ Add the sweet potatoes and rice and sauté for about 3 minutes.

⇒ Add the broth, salt, and pepper and boil. Simmer within 30 to 40 minutes.

⇒ Combine in the lemon juice and parsley, then serve.

Nutrition: Calories 425 Fat: 15g Total Carbohydrates: 65g Sugar: 6g Fiber: 6gProtein: 11gSodium: 1045mg

33) Baked Tilapia Recipe With Pecan Rosemary Topping

Preparation Time: **Cooking Time: 20 Minutes**   **Servings:4**

Ingredients:

- 4 tilapia fillets (4 ounces each)
- ½ teaspoon brown sugar or coconut palm sugar
- 2 teaspoons fresh rosemary, chopped
- 1/3 cup raw pecans, chopped
- A pinch of cayenne pepper
- 1 ½ teaspoon olive oil
- 1 large egg white
- 1/8 teaspoon salt
- 1/3 cup panko breadcrumbs, preferably whole-wheat

Directions:

⇒ Heat-up your oven to 350 F.

⇒ Stir the pecans with breadcrumbs, coconut palm sugar, rosemary, cayenne pepper, and salt in a small-sized baking dish. Add the olive oil; toss.

⇒ Bake within 7 to 8 minutes, until the mixture turns light golden brown.

⇒ Adjust the heat to 400 F and coat a large-sized glass baking dish with some cooking spray.

⇒ Whisk the egg white in the shallow dish. Work in batches; dip the fish (one tilapia at a time) into the egg white, and then, coating lightly into the pecan mixture. Put the coated fillets in the baking dish.

⇒ Press the leftover pecan mixture over the tilapia fillets.

⇒ Bake within 8 to 10 minutes. Serve immediately & enjoy.

Nutrition: Kcal 222 Fat: 10 g Fiber: 2 g Protein: 27 g

34) Black Bean Tortilla Wrap

Preparation Time: **Cooking Time: 0 Minutes**   **Servings:2**

Ingredients:

- ¼ cup of corn
- 1 handful of fresh basil
- ½ cup of arugula
- 1 tablespoon of nutritional yeast
- ¼ cup of canned black beans
- 1 peach, sliced
- 1 teaspoon of lime juice
- 2 gluten-free tortillas

Directions:

⇒ Divide the beans, corn, arugula, and peaches between the two tortillas.

⇒ Top each tortilla with half the fresh basil and lime juice

Nutrition: Total Carbohydrates 44g Dietary Fiber: 7g Protein: 8g Total Fat: 1g Calories: 203

35) White Bean Chicken With Winter Green Vegetables

Preparation Time: **Cooking Time: 45 Minutes**   **Servings:8**

Ingredients:

- 4 Garlic cloves
- 1tbsp Olive oil
- 3 medium parsnips
- 1kg Small cubes of chicken
- 1 Teaspoon cumin powder
- 2 Leaks & 1 Green part
- 2 Carrots (cut into cubes)
- 1 ¼ White kidney beans (overnight soaked)
- ½ Teaspoon dried oregano
- 2 Teaspoon Kosher salt
- Cilantro leaves
- 1 1/2tbsp Ground ancho chilies

Directions:

⇒ Cook garlic, leeks, chicken, and olive oil in a large pot on a medium flame for 5 minutes.

⇒ Now add carrots and parsnips, and after stirring for 2 minutes, add all seasoning ingredients.

⇒ Stir until the fragrant starts coming from it.

⇒ Now add beans and 5 cups of water in the pot.

⇒ Bring it to a boil and reduce the flame.

⇒ Allow it to simmer almost for 30 minutes and garnish with parsley and cilantro leaves.

Nutrition: Calories 263Carbs: 24gFat: 7g Protein: 26g

36) Herbed Baked Salmon

Preparation Time: **Cooking Time: 15 Minutes**   **Servings:2**

Ingredients:

- 10 oz. Salmon Fillet
- 1 tsp. Olive Oil
- 1 tsp. Honey
- 1 tsp. Tarragon, fresh

- 1/8 tsp. Salt
- 2 tsp. Dijon Mustard
- ¼ tsp. Thyme, dried
- ¼ tsp. Oregano, dried

Directions:

⇒ Preheat the oven to 425 ° F.

⇒ After that, combine all the ingredients, excluding the salmon in a medium-sized bowl.

⇒ Now, spoon this mixture evenly over the salmon.

⇒ Then, place the salmon with the skin side down on the parchment paper-lined baking sheet.

⇒ Finally, bake for 8 minutes or until the fish flakes.

Nutrition: Calories: 239KcalProteins: 31gCarbohydrates: 3gFat: 11g

37) Valencia Salad

Preparation Time: **Cooking Time: 0 Minutes**   **Servings:10**

Ingredients:

- 1 tsp. Kalamata olives in oil, pitted, drained lightly, halved, julienned
- 1 head, small Romaine lettuce, rinsed, spun-dried, sliced into bite-sized pieces
- ½ piece, small shallot, julienned
- 1 tsp. Dijon mustard
- ½ small satsuma or tangerine, pulp only

- 1 tsp. white wine vinegar
- 1 tsp. extra virgin olive oil
- 1 pinch fresh thyme, minced
- Pinch of sea salt
- Pinch of black pepper, to taste

Directions:

⇒ Combine vinegar, oil, fresh thyme, salt, mustard, black pepper, and honey, if using. Whisk well until dressing emulsifies a little.

⇒ Toss together the remaining salad ingredients in a salad bowl.

⇒ Drizzle dressing on top when about to serve. Serve immediately with 1 slice if sugar-free sourdough bread or saltine.

Nutrition: Calories 238Carbs: 23gFat: 15gProtein: 8g

38) "eat Your Greens" Soup

Preparation Time: **Cooking Time: 20 Minutes**   **Servings:4**

Ingredients:

- ¼ cup extra-virgin olive oil
- 2 leeks, white parts only, thinly sliced
- 1 fennel bulb, trimmed and thinly sliced
- 1 garlic clove, peeled
- 1 bunch Swiss chard, coarsely chopped
- 4 cups coarsely chopped kale

- 4 cups coarsely chopped mustard greens
- 3 cups vegetable broth
- 2 tablespoons apple cider vinegar
- 1 teaspoon salt
- ¼ teaspoon freshly ground black pepper
- ¼ cup chopped cashews (optional)

Directions:

⇒ Heat-up the oil over high heat in a large pot.

⇒ Add the leeks, fennel, and garlic and sauté until softened, for about 5 minutes.

⇒ Add the Swiss chard, kale, and mustard greens and sauté until the greens wilt, 2 to 3 minutes.

⇒ Put the broth and boil.

⇒ Simmer within 5 minutes.

⇒ Stir in the vinegar, salt, pepper, and cashews (if using).

⇒ Purée the soup using an immersion blender until smooth and serve.

Nutrition: Calories 238 Total Fat: 14g Total Carbohydrates: 22g Sugar: 4g Fiber: 6gProtein: 9gSodium: 1294mg

39)Miso Salmon And Green Beans

Preparation Time: **Cooking Time: 25 Minutes** **Servings:4**

Ingredients:

- 1 tablespoon sesame oil
- 1-pound green beans, trimmed
- 1-pound skin-on salmon fillets, cut into 4 steaks
- ¼ cup white miso
- 2 teaspoons gluten-free tamari or soy sauce
- 2 scallions, thinly sliced

Directions:

⇒ Preheat the oven to 400°F. Grease the baking sheet with the oil.

⇒ Put the green beans, then the salmon on top of the green beans, and brush each piece with the miso.

⇒ Roast within 20 to 25 minutes.

⇒ Drizzle with the tamari, sprinkle with the scallions, and serve.

Nutrition: Calories 213 Total Fat: 7g Total Carbohydrates: 13g Sugar: 3g Fiber: 5g Protein: 27g Sodium: 989mg

40)Leek, Chicken, And Spinach Soup

Preparation Time: **Cooking Time: 15 Minutes** **Servings:4**

Ingredients:

- 3 tablespoons unsalted butter
- 2 leeks, white parts only, thinly sliced
- 4 cups baby spinach
- 4 cups chicken broth
- 1 teaspoon salt
- ¼ teaspoon freshly ground black pepper
- 2 cups shredded rotisserie chicken
- 1 tablespoon thinly sliced fresh chives
- 2 teaspoons grated or minced lemon zest

Directions:

⇒ Dissolve the butter over high heat in a large pot.

⇒ Add the leeks and sauté until softened and beginning to brown, 3 to 5 minutes.

⇒ Add the spinach, broth, salt, and pepper and boil.

⇒ Simmer within 1 to 2 minutes.

⇒ Put the chicken and cook within 1 to 2 minutes.

⇒ Sprinkle with the chives and lemon zest and serve.

Nutrition: Calories 256 Total Fat: 12g Total Carbohydrates: 9g Sugar: 3g Fiber: 2gProtein: 27gSodium: 1483mg

41)Dark Choco Bombs

Preparation Time: **Cooking Time: 5 Minutes** **Servings:24**

Ingredients:

- 1 cup heavy cream
- 1 cup cream cheese softened
- 1 teaspoon vanilla essence
- 1/2 cup dark chocolate
- 2 oz. Stevia

Directions:

⇒ Melt chocolate in a bowl by heating in a microwave.

⇒ Beat the rest of the ingredients in a mixer until fluffy, then stir in the chocolate melt.

⇒ Mix well, then divide the mixture in a muffin tray lined with muffin cups.

⇒ Refrigerate for 3 hrs.

⇒ Serve.

Nutrition: Calories 97 Fat 5 g, Carbs 1 g, Protein 1 g, Fiber 0 g

42) Italian Stuffed Peppers

Preparation Time: **Cooking Time: 40 Minutes**   **Servings:6**

Ingredients:

- 1 teaspoon garlic powder
- 1/2 cup mozzarella, shredded
- 1 lb. lean ground meat
- 1/2 cup parmesan cheese
- 3 bell peppers, cut into half lengthwise, stems, seeds and ribs removed

- 1 (10 oz.) package frozen spinach
- 2 cups marinara sauce
- 1/2 teaspoon salt
- 1 teaspoon Italian seasoning

Directions:

⇒ Coat a foil-lined baking sheet with non-stick spray. Place the peppers on the baking pan.

⇒ Add turkey to a non-stick pan and cook over medium heat until no longer pink.

⇒ When almost cooked, add 2 cups of marinara sauce and seasonings—Cook for about 8-10 minutes.

⇒ Add spinach along with 1/2 cup parmesan cheese. Stir until well-combined.

⇒ Add half cup of the meat mixture into each pepper and divide cheese among all—Preheat the oven to 450 F.

⇒ Bake peppers for about 25-30 minutes. Cool, and serve.

Nutrition: 150 calories 2 g fat 11 g total carbs 20 g protein

43) Smoked Trout Wrapped In Lettuce

Preparation Time: **Cooking Time: 45 Minutes**   **Servings:4**

Ingredients:

- ¼ Cup salt-roasted potatoes
- 1 cup grape tomatoes
- ½ Cup basil leaves
- 16 small & medium size lettuce leaves
- 1/3 cup Asian sweet chili
- 2 Carrots

- 1/3 Cup Shallots (thin sliced)
- ¼ Cup thin slice Jalapenos
- 1tbsp Sugar
- 2-4.5 Ounces skinless smoked trout
- 2tbsp Fresh lime Juice
- 1 Cucumber

Directions:

⇒ Cut carrots and cucumber in slim strip size.

⇒ Marinate these vegetables for 20 mins with sugar, fish sauce, lime juice, shallots, and jalapeno.

⇒ Add trout pieces and other herbs in this vegetable mixture and blend.

⇒ Strain water from vegetable and trout mixture and again toss it to blend.

⇒ Place lettuce leaves on a plate and transfer trout salad on them.

⇒ Garnish this salad with peanuts and chili sauce.

Nutrition: Calories 180Carbs: 0gFat: 12gProtein: 18g

Chapter 4: Fish & Seafood Recipes

44) Broiled Sea Bass

Preparation Time: **Cooking Time:**   **Servings:2**

Ingredients:

- 2 minced garlic cloves
- Pepper.
- 1 tbsp. lemon juice

- 2 white sea bass fillets
- ¼ tsp. herb seasoning blend

Directions:

⇒ Spray a broiler pan with some olive oil and place the fillets on it.

⇒ Sprinkle the lemon juice, garlic and the spices over the fillets.

⇒ Broil for about 10 min or until the fish is golden.

⇒ Serve over a bed of sautéed spinach if desired.

Nutrition: Calories: 169, Fat:9.3 g, Carbs:0.34 g, Protein:15.3 g, Sugars:0.2 g, Sodium:323 mg

45) Spicy Cod

Preparation Time: **Cooking Time:**   **Servings:4**

Ingredients:

- 2 tbsps. Fresh chopped parsley
- 2 lbs. cod fillets

- 2 c. low sodium salsa
- 1 tbsp. flavorless oil

Directions:

⇒ Preheat the oven to 350∘F.

⇒ In a large, deep baking dish drizzle the oil along the bottom. Place the cod fillets in the dish. Pour the salsa over the fish. Cover with foil for 20 minutes. Remove the foil last 10 minutes of cooking.

⇒ Bake in the oven for 20 – 30 minutes, until the fish is flaky.

⇒ Serve with white or brown rice. Garnish with parsley.

Nutrition: Calories: 110, Fat:11 g, Carbs:83 g, Protein:16.5 g, Sugars:0 g, Sodium:122 mg

46) Smoked Trout Spread

Preparation Time: **Cooking Time:**   **Servings:2**

Ingredients:

- 2 tsps. Fresh lemon juice
- ½ c. low-fat cottage cheese
- 1 diced celery stalk
- ¼ lb. skinned smoked trout fillet,

- ½ tsp. Worcestershire sauce
- 1 tsp. hot pepper sauce
- ¼ c. coarsely chopped red onion

Directions:

⇒ Combine the trout, cottage cheese, red onion, lemon juice, hot pepper sauce and Worcestershire sauce in a blender or food processor.

⇒ Process until smooth, stopping to scrape down the sides of the bowl as needed.

⇒ Fold in the diced celery.

⇒ Keep in an air-tight container in the refrigerator.

Nutrition: Calories: 57, Fat:4 g, Carbs:1 g, Protein:4 g, Sugars:0 g, Sodium:660 mg

47) Tuna And Shallots

Preparation Time: **Cooking Time:**   **Servings:4**

Ingredients:

- ½ c. low-sodium chicken stock
- 1 tbsp. olive oil
- 4 boneless and skinless tuna fillets
- 2 chopped shallots

- 1 tsp. sweet paprika
- 2 tbsps. lime juice
- ¼ tsp. black pepper

Directions:

⇒ Heat up a pan with the oil over medium-high heat, add shallots and sauté for 3 minutes.

⇒ Add the fish and cook it for 4 minutes on each side.

⇒ Add the rest of the ingredients, cook everything for 3 minutes more, divide between plates and serve.

Nutrition: Calories: 4040, Fat:34.6 g, Carbs:3 g, Protein:21.4 g, Sugars:0.5 g, Sodium:1000 mg

48) Hot Tuna Steak

Preparation Time: **Cooking Time:**   **Servings:6**

Ingredients:

- 2 tbsps. Fresh lemon juice
- Pepper.
- Roasted orange garlic mayonnaise
- ¼ c. whole black peppercorns

- 6 sliced tuna steaks
- 2 tbsps. Extra-virgin olive oil
- Salt

Directions:

⇒ Place the tuna in a bowl to fit. Add the oil, lemon juice, salt and pepper. Turn the tuna to coat well in the marinade. Let rest 15 to 20 minutes, turning once.

⇒ Place the peppercorns in a double thickness of plastic bags. Tap the peppercorns with a heavy saucepan or small mallet to crush them coarsely. Place on a large plate.

⇒ When ready to cook the tuna, dip the edges into the crushed peppercorns. Heat a nonstick skillet over medium heat. Sear the tuna steaks, in batches if necessary, for 4 minutes per side for medium-rare fish, adding 2 to 3 tablespoons of the marinade to the skillet if necessary, to prevent sticking.

⇒ Serve dolloped with roasted orange garlic mayonnaise

Nutrition: Calories: 124, Fat:0.4 g, Carbs:0.6 g, Protein:28 g, Sugars:0 g, Sodium:77 mg

Chapter 5: Meat Recipes

49) Roast Chicken Dal

Preparation Time: **Cooking Time:**   Servings: 4

Ingredients:

- 15 oz. rinsed lentils
- ¼ c. low-fat plain yogurt
- 1 minced small onion
- 4 c. de-boned, skinless and roasted chicken
- 2 tsps. Curry powder
- 1 ½ tsps. Canola oil
- 14 oz. fire-roasted diced tomatoes
- ¼ tsp. salt

Directions:

⇒ Heat oil in a large heavy saucepan over medium-high heat.

⇒ Add onion and cook, stirring, until softened but not browned, 3 to 4 minutes.

⇒ Add curry powder and cook, stirring, until combined with the onion and intensely aromatic, 20 to 30 seconds.

⇒ Stir in lentils, tomatoes, chicken and salt and cook, stirring often, until heated through.

⇒ Remove from the heat and stir in yogurt. Serve immediately.

Nutrition: Calories: 307, Fat:6 g, Carbs:30 g, Protein:35 g, Sugars:0.1 g, Sodium:361 mg

50) Oregano Pork

Preparation Time: **Cooking Time: 8 Hours**   Servings: 4

Ingredients:

- 2 pounds pork roast, sliced
- 2 tablespoons oregano, chopped
- ¼ cup balsamic vinegar
- 1 cup tomato paste
- 1 tablespoon sweet paprika
- 1 teaspoon onion powder
- 2 tablespoons chili powder
- 2 garlic cloves, minced
- A pinch of salt and black pepper

Directions:

⇒ In your slow cooker, combine the roast with the oregano, the vinegar and the other ingredients, toss, put the lid on and cook on Low for 8 hours.

⇒ Divide everything between plates and serve.

Nutrition: calories 300, fat 5, fiber 2, carbs 12, protein 24

51) Chicken And Avocado Bake

Preparation Time: **Cooking Time:**   Servings: 4

Ingredients:

- 2 thinly sliced green onion stalks
- Mashed avocado
- 170 g non-fat Greek yogurt
- 1 ¼ g salt
- 4 chicken breasts
- 15 g blackened seasoning

Directions:

⇒ Start by putting your chicken breast in a plastic zip lock bag with the blackened seasoning. Close and shake, then marinate for about 2-5 minutes.

⇒ As your chicken is marinating, go ahead and put your Greek Yogurt, mashed avocado, and salt in your blender and pulse until smooth.

⇒ Place a large skillet or cast-iron pan on the stove at medium heat, oil the pan and cook the chicken until it is cooked through. You'll need about 5 minutes on each side. However, try not to dry the juices and plate it as soon as the meat is cooked.

⇒ Top with the yogurt mixture.

Nutrition: Calories: 296, Fat:13.5 g, Carbs:6.6 g, Protein:35.37 g, Sugars:0.8 g, Sodium:173 mg

52) Five-spice Roasted Duck Breasts

Preparation Time:	Cooking Time:	Servings:4

Ingredients:

- 1 tsp. five-spice powder
- ¼ tsp. cornstarch
- 2 orange juice and zest
- 1 tbsp. reduced-sodium soy sauce
- 2 lbs. de-boned duck breast
- ½ tsp. kosher salt
- 2 tsps. Honey

Directions:

⇒ Preheat oven to 375 0F.

⇒ Place duck skin-side down on a cutting board. Trim off all excess skin that hangs over the sides. Turnover and make three parallel, diagonal cuts in the skin of each breast, cutting through the fat but not into the meat. Sprinkle both sides with five-spice powder and salt.

⇒ Place the duck skin-side down in an ovenproof skillet over medium-low heat.

⇒ Cook until the fat is melted and the skin is golden brown, about 10 minutes. Transfer the duck to a plate; pour off all the fat from the pan. Return the duck to the pan skin-side up and transfer to the oven.

⇒ Roast the duck for 10 to 15 minutes for medium, depending on the size of the breast, until a thermometer inserted into the thickest part registers 150 0F.

⇒ Transfer to a cutting board; let rest for 5 minutes.

⇒ Pour off any fat remaining in the pan (take care, the handle will still be hot); place the pan over medium-high heat and add orange juice and honey. Bring to a simmer, stirring to scrape up any browned bits.

⇒ Add orange zest and soy sauce and continue to cook until the sauce is slightly reduced, about 1 minute. Stir cornstarch mixture then whisk into the sauce; cook, stirring, until slightly thickened, 1 minute.

⇒ Remove the duck skin and thinly slice the breast meat. Drizzle with the orange sauce.

Nutrition: Calories: 152, Fat:2 g, Carbs:8 g, Protein:24 g, Sugars:5 g, Sodium:309 mg

53) Pork Chops With Tomato Salsa

Preparation Time:	Cooking Time: 15 Minutes	Servings:4

Ingredients:

- 4 pork chops
- 1 tablespoon olive oil
- 4 scallions, chopped
- 1 teaspoon cumin, ground
- ½ tablespoon hot paprika
- 1 teaspoon garlic powder
- A pinch of sea salt and black pepper
- 1 small red onion, chopped
- 2 tomatoes, cubed
- 2 tablespoons lime juice
- 1 jalapeno, chopped
- ¼ cup cilantro, chopped
- 1 tablespoon lime juice

Directions:

⇒ Heat up a pan with the oil over medium heat, add the scallions and sauté for 5 minutes.

⇒ Add the meat, cumin paprika, garlic powder, salt and pepper, toss, cook for 5 minutes on each side and divide between plates.

⇒ In a bowl, combine the tomatoes with the remaining ingredients, toss, divide next to the pork chops and serve.

Nutrition: calories 313, fat 23.7, fiber 1.7, carbs 5.9, protein 19.2

54) Tuscan Chicken With Tomatoes, Olives, And Zucchini

Preparation Time:	Cooking Time: 20 Minutes	Servings:4

Ingredients:

- 4 boneless, skinless chicken breast halves, pounded to ½- to ¾-inch thickness
- 1 teaspoon garlic powder
- ½ teaspoon sea salt
- ⅛ teaspoon freshly ground black pepper
- 2 tablespoons extra-virgin olive oil

- 2 cups cherry tomatoes
- ½ cup sliced green olives
- 1 zucchini, chopped
- ¼ cup dry white wine

Directions:

⇒ On a clean work surface, rub the chicken breasts with garlic powder, salt, and ground black pepper.

⇒ Heat the olive oil in a nonstick skillet over medium-high heat until shimmering.

⇒ Add the chicken and cook for 16 minutes or until the internal temperature reaches at least 165°F (74°C). Flip the chicken halfway through the cooking time. Transfer to a large plate and cover with aluminum foil to keep warm.

⇒ Add the tomatoes, olives, and zucchini to the skillet and sauté for 4 minutes or until the vegetables are soft.

⇒ Add the white wine to the skillet and simmer for 1 minutes.

⇒ Remove the aluminum foil and top the chicken with the vegetables and their juices, then serve warm.

Nutrition: calories: 172 ; fat: 11.1g ; protein: 8.2g ; carbs: 7.9g ; fiber: 2.1g ; sugar: 4.2g ; sodium: 742mg

55) Pork Salad

Preparation Time:	Cooking Time: 10 Minutes	Servings:4

Ingredients:

- 1-pound pork stew meat, cut into strips
- 3 tablespoons olive oil
- 4 scallions, chopped
- 2 tablespoons lemon juice
- 2 tablespoons balsamic vinegar

- 2 cups mixed salad greens
- 1 avocado, peeled, pitted and roughly cubed
- 1 cucumber, sliced
- 2 tomatoes, cubed
- A pinch of salt and black pepper

Directions:

⇒ Heat up a pan with 2 tablespoons of oil over medium heat, add the scallions, the meat and the lemon juice, toss and cook for 10 minutes.

⇒ In a salad bowl, combine the salad greens with the meat and the remaining ingredients, toss and serve.

Nutrition: calories 225, fat 6.4, fiber 4, carbs 8, protein 11

56) Lime Pork And Green Beans

Preparation Time:	Cooking Time: 40 Minutes	Servings:4

Ingredients:

- 2 pounds pork stew meat, cubed
- 2 tablespoons avocado oil
- ½ cup green beans, trimmed and halved
- 2 tablespoons lime juice

- 1 cup coconut milk
- 1 tablespoon rosemary, chopped
- A pinch of salt and black pepper

Directions:

⇒ Heat up a pan with the oil over medium heat, add the meat and brown for 5 minutes.

⇒ Add the rest of the ingredients, toss gently, bring to a simmer and cook over medium heat for 35 minutes more.

⇒ Divide the mix between plates and serve.

Nutrition: calories 260, fat 5, fiber 8, carbs 9, protein 13

57) Pork With Chili Zucchinis And Tomatoes

Preparation Time: **Cooking Time: 35 Minutes**   **Servings:4**

Ingredients:

- 2 tomatoes, cubed
- 2 pounds pork stew meat, cubed
- 4 scallions, chopped
- 2 tablespoons olive oil
- 1 zucchini, sliced

- Juice of 1 lime
- 2 tablespoons chili powder
- ½ tablespoons cumin powder
- A pinch of sea salt and black pepper

Directions:

⇒ Heat up a pan with the oil over medium heat, add the scallions and sauté for 5 minutes.

⇒ Add the meat and brown for 5 minutes more.

⇒ Add the tomatoes and the other ingredients, toss, cook over medium heat for 25 minutes more, divide between plates and serve.

Nutrition: calories 300, fat 5, fiber 2, carbs 12, protein 14

58) Pork With Olives

Preparation Time: **Cooking Time: 40 Minutes**   **Servings:4**

Ingredients:

- 1 yellow onion, chopped
- 4 pork chops
- 2 tablespoons olive oil
- 1 tablespoon sweet paprika
- 2 tablespoons balsamic vinegar

- ¼ cup kalamata olives, pitted and chopped
- 1 tablespoon cilantro, chopped
- A pinch of sea salt and black pepper

Directions:

⇒ Heat up a pan with the oil over medium heat, add the onion and sauté for 5 minutes.

⇒ Add the meat and brown for 5 minutes more.

⇒ Add the rest of the ingredients, toss, cook over medium heat for 30 minutes, divide between plates and serve.

Nutrition: calories 280, fat 11, fiber 6, carbs 10, protein 21

59) Pork With Nutmeg Squash

Preparation Time: **Cooking Time: 35 Minutes**   **Servings:4**

Ingredients:

- 1-pound pork stew meat, cubed
- 1 butternut squash, peeled and cubed
- 1 yellow onion, chopped
- 2 tablespoons olive oil
- 2 garlic cloves, minced

- ½ teaspoon garam masala
- ½ teaspoon nutmeg, ground
- 1 teaspoon chili flakes, crushed
- 1 tablespoon balsamic vinegar
- A pinch of sea salt and black pepper

Directions:

⇒ Heat up a pan with the oil over medium-high heat, add the onion and the garlic and sauté for 5 minutes.

⇒ Add the meat and brown for another 5 minutes.

⇒ Add the rest of the ingredients, toss, cook over medium heat for 25 minutes, divide between plates and serve.

Nutrition: calories 348, fat 18.2, fiber 2.1, carbs 11.4, protein 34.3

60) Creamy Pork And Tomatoes

Preparation Time: **Cooking Time: 35 Minutes**   **Servings:4**

Ingredients:

- 2 pounds pork stew meat, cubed
- 2 tablespoons avocado oil
- 1 cup tomatoes, cubed
- 1 cup coconut cream
- 1 tablespoon mint, chopped

- 1 jalapeno pepper, chopped
- A pinch of sea salt and black pepper
- 1 tablespoon hot pepper
- 2 tablespoons lemon juice

Directions:

⇒ Heat up a pan with the oil over medium heat, add the meat and brown for 5 minutes.

⇒ Add the rest of the ingredients, toss, cook over medium heat for 30 minutes more, divide between plates and serve.

Nutrition: calories 230, fat 4, fiber 6, carbs 9, protein 14

61) Lemon Tenderloin

Preparation Time: **Cooking Time: 25 Minutes**   **Servings:2**

Ingredients:

- ¼ teaspoon za'atar seasoning
- Zest of 1 lemon
- ½ teaspoon dried thyme
- ¼ teaspoon garlic powder

- ¼ teaspoon salt
- 1 tablespoon olive oil
- 1 (8-ounce / 227-g) pork tenderloin, sliver skin trimmed

Directions:

⇒ Preheat the oven to 425°F (220°C).

⇒ Combine the za'atar seasoning, lemon zest, thyme, garlic powder, and salt in a bowl, then rub the pork tenderloin with the mixture on both sides.

⇒ Warm the olive oil in an oven-safe skillet over medium-high heat until shimmering.

⇒ Add the pork tenderloin and sear for 6 minutes or until browned. Flip the pork halfway through the cooking time.

⇒ Arrange the skillet in the preheated oven and roast for 15 minutes or until an instant-read thermometer inserted in the thickest part of the tenderloin registers at least 145°F (63°C).

⇒ Transfer the cooked tenderloin to a large plate and allow to cool for a few minutes before serving.

Nutrition: calories: 184 ; fat: 10.8g ; carbs: 1.2g ; fiber: 0g ; protein: 20.1g ; sodium: 358mg

62) Chicken With Broccoli

Preparation Time: **Cooking Time:**   **Servings:4**

Ingredients:

- 1 chopped small white onion
- 1½ c. low-fat, low-sodium chicken broth
- Freshly ground black pepper

- 2 c. chopped broccoli
- 1 lb. cubed, skinless and de-boned chicken thighs
- 2 minced garlic cloves

Directions:

⇒ In a slow cooker, add all ingredients and mix well.

⇒ Set slow cooker on low.

⇒ Cover and cook for 4-5 hours.

⇒ Serve hot.

Nutrition: Calories: 300, Fat:9 g, Carbs:19 g, Protein:31 g, Sugars:6 g, Sodium:200 mg

63) Pork With Mushrooms And Cucumbers

Preparation Time: **Cooking Time: 25 Minutes**   **Servings:4**

Ingredients:

- 2 tablespoons olive oil
- ½ teaspoon oregano, dried
- 4 pork chops
- 2 garlic cloves, minced
- Juice of 1 lime

- ¼ cup cilantro, chopped
- A pinch of sea salt and black pepper
- 1 cup white mushrooms, halved
- 2 tablespoons balsamic vinegar

Directions:

⇒ Heat up a pan with the oil over medium heat, add the pork chops and brown for 2 minutes on each side.

⇒ Add the rest of the ingredients, toss, cook over medium heat for 20 minutes, divide between plates and serve.

Nutrition: calories 220, fat 6, fiber 8, carbs 14.2, protein 20

64) Chicken Chopstick

Preparation Time: **Cooking Time:**   **Servings:4**

Ingredients:

- ¼ c. diced chopped onion
- 1 pack cooked chow Mein noodles
- Fresh ground pepper
- 2 cans cream mushroom soup

- 1 ¼ c. sliced celery
- 1 c. cashew nuts
- 2 c. cubed cooked chicken
- ½ c. water

Directions:

⇒ 1 ¼ c. sliced celery

⇒ 1 c. cashew nuts

⇒ 2 c. cubed cooked chicken

⇒ ½ c. water

⇒ Add half the noodles to the mixture, stir until coated.

⇒ Top the casserole with the rest of the noodles.

⇒ Place the pot in the oven. Bake for 25 minutes.

⇒ Serve immediately.

Nutrition: Calories: 201, Fat:17 g, Carbs:15 g, Protein:13 g, Sugars:7 g, Sodium:10 mg

65) Balsamic Roast Chicken

Preparation Time: **Cooking Time:**   **Servings:4**

Ingredients:

- 1 tbsp. minced fresh rosemary
- 1 minced garlic clove
- Black pepper
- 1 tbsp. olive oil

- 1 tsp. brown sugar
- 6 rosemary sprigs
- 1 whole chicken
- ½ c. balsamic vinegar

Directions:

⇒ Combine garlic, minced rosemary, black pepper and the olive oil. Rub the chicken with the herbal olive oil mixture.

⇒ Put 3 rosemary sprigs into the chicken cavity.

⇒ Place the chicken into a roasting pan and roast at 400F for about 1 hr. 30 minutes.

⇒ When the chicken is golden and the juices run clear, transfer to a serving dish.

⇒ In a saucepan dissolve the sugar in balsamic vinegar over heat. Do not boil.

⇒ Carve the chicken and top with vinegar mixture.

Nutrition: Calories: 587, Fat:37.8 g, Carbs:2.5 g, Protein:54.1 g, Sugars:0 g, Sodium:600 mg

66) Peach Chicken Treat

Preparation Time: **Cooking Time:**   **Servings: 4-5**

Ingredients:

- 2 minced garlic cloves
- ¼ c. balsamic vinegar
- 4 sliced peaches
- 4 skinless, deboned chicken breasts

- ¼ c. chopped basil
- 1 tbsp. olive oil
- 1 chopped shallot
- ¼ tsp. black pepper

Directions:

⇒ Heat up the oil in a saucepan over medium-high flame.

⇒ Add the meat and season with black pepper; fry for 8 minutes on each side and set aside to rest in a plate.

⇒ In the same pan, add the shallot and garlic; stir and cook for 2 minutes.

⇒ Add the peaches; stir and cook for 4-5 more minutes.

⇒ Add the vinegar, cooked chicken, and basil; toss and simmer covered for 3-4 minutes more.

⇒ Serve warm.

Nutrition: Calories: 270, Fat:0 g, Carbs:6.6 g, Protein:1.5 g, Sugars:24 g, Sodium:87 mg

67) Ground Pork Pan

Preparation Time: **Cooking Time: 15 Minutes**   **Servings:4**

Ingredients:

- 2 garlic cloves, minced
- 2 red chilies, chopped
- 2 tablespoons olive oil
- 2 pounds pork stew meat, ground
- 1 red bell pepper, chopped
- 1 green bell pepper, chopped

- 1 tomato, cubed
- ½ cup mushrooms, halved
- A pinch of sea salt and black pepper
- 1 tablespoon basil, chopped
- 2 tablespoons coconut aminos

Directions:

⇒ Heat up a pan with the oil over medium heat, add the garlic, chilies, bell peppers, tomato and the mushrooms and sauté for 5 minutes.

⇒ Add the meat and the rest of the ingredients, toss, cook over medium heat for 10 minutes more, divide between plates and serve.

Nutrition: calories 200, fat 3, fiber 5, carbs 7, protein 17

68) Parsley Pork And Artichokes

Preparation Time: **Cooking Time: 35 Minutes**   **Servings:4**

Ingredients:

- 2 tablespoons balsamic vinegar
- 1 cup canned artichoke hearts, drained and quartered
- 2 tablespoons olive oil
- 2 pounds pork stew meat, cubed
- 2 tablespoons parsley, chopped

- 1 teaspoon cumin, ground
- 1 teaspoon turmeric powder
- 2 garlic cloves, minced
- A pinch of sea salt and black pepper

Directions:

⇒ Heat up a pan with the oil over medium heat, add the meat and brown for 5 minutes.

⇒ Add the artichokes, the vinegar and the other ingredients, toss, cook over medium heat for 30 minutes, divide between plates and serve.

Nutrition: calories 260, fat 5, fiber 4, carbs 11, protein 20

69) Pork With Thyme Sweet Potatoes

Preparation Time: **Cooking Time: 35 Minutes**   **Servings:4**

Ingredients:

- 2 sweet potatoes, peeled and cut into wedges
- 4 pork chops
- 3 spring onions, chopped
- 1 tablespoon thyme, chopped
- 2 tablespoons olive oil
- 4 garlic cloves, minced
- A pinch of sea salt and black pepper
- ½ cup vegetable stock
- ½ tablespoon chives, chopped

Directions:

⇒ In a roasting pan, combine the pork chops with the potatoes and the other ingredients, toss gently and cook at 390 degrees F for 35 minutes.

⇒ Divide everything between plates and serve.

Nutrition: calories 210, fat 12.2, fiber 5.2, carbs 12, protein 10

70) Curry Pork Mix

Preparation Time: **Cooking Time: 30 Minutes**   **Servings:4**

Ingredients:

- 2 tablespoon olive oil
- 4 scallions, chopped
- 2 garlic cloves, minced
- 2 pounds pork stew meat, cubed
- 2 tablespoons red curry paste
- 1 teaspoon chili paste
- 2 tablespoons balsamic vinegar
- ¼ cup vegetable stock
- ¼ cup parsley, chopped

Directions:

⇒ Heat up a pan with the oil over medium-high heat, add the scallions and the garlic and sauté for 5 minutes.

⇒ Add the meat and brown for 5 minutes more.

⇒ Add the remaining ingredients, toss, cook over medium heat for 20 minutes, divide between plates and serve.

Nutrition: calories 220, fat 3, fiber 4, carbs 7, protein 12

71) Stir-fried Chicken And Broccoli

Preparation Time: **Cooking Time: 10 Minutes**   **Servings:4**

Ingredients:

- 3 tablespoons extra-virgin olive oil
- 1½ cups broccoli florets
- 1½ pounds (680 g) boneless, skinless chicken breasts, cut into bite-size pieces
- ½ onion, chopped
- ½ teaspoon sea salt
- ⅛ teaspoon freshly ground black pepper
- 3 garlic cloves, minced
- 2 cups cooked brown rice

Directions:

⇒ Heat the olive oil in a large nonstick skillet over medium-high heat until shimmering.

⇒ Add the broccoli, chicken, and onion to the skillet and stir well. Season with sea salt and black pepper.

⇒ Stir-fry for about 8 minutes, or until the chicken is golden browned and cooked through.

⇒ Toss in the garlic and cook for 30 seconds, stirring constantly, or until the garlic is fragrant.

⇒ Remove from the heat to a plate and serve over the cooked brown rice.

Nutrition: calories: 344 ; fat: 14.1g ; protein: 14.1g ; carbs: 40.9g ; fiber: 3.2g ; sugar: 1.2g ; sodium: 275mg

72) Chicken And Broccoli

Preparation Time: **Cooking Time:**   **Servings:4**

Ingredients:

- 2 minced garlic cloves
- 4 de-boned, skinless chicken breasts
- ½ c. coconut cream
- 1 tbsp. chopped oregano

- 2 c. broccoli florets
- 1 tbsp. organic olive oil
- 1 c. chopped red onions

Directions:

⇒ Heat up a pan while using the oil over medium-high heat, add chicken breasts and cook for 5 minutes on each side.

⇒ Add onions and garlic, stir and cook for 5 minutes more.

⇒ Add oregano, broccoli and cream, toss everything, cook for ten minutes more, divide between plates and serve.

⇒ Enjoy!

Nutrition: Calories: 287, Fat:10 g, Carbs:14 g, Protein:19 g, Sugars:10 g, Sodium:1106 mg

73) Pork With Cabbage And Kale

Preparation Time: **Cooking Time: 35 Minutes**   **Servings:4**

Ingredients:

- 1-pound pork stew meat, cut into strips
- 2 tablespoons olive oil
- 1 yellow onion, chopped
- A pinch of sea salt and black pepper
- cup green cabbage, shredded

- ½ cup baby kale
- 2 tablespoons oregano, dried
- 2 tablespoons balsamic vinegar
- ¼ cup vegetable stock

Directions:

⇒ Heat up a pan with the oil over medium-high heat, add the onion and the meat and brown for 5 minutes.

⇒ Add the cabbage and the other ingredients, toss gently and bake everything at 390 degrees F for 30 minutes.

⇒ Divide the whole mix between plates and serve.

Nutrition: calories 331, fat 18.7, fiber 2.1, carbs 6.5, protein 34.2

74) Mediterranean Chicken Bake With Vegetables

Preparation Time: **Cooking Time: 20 Minutes**   **Servings:4**

Ingredients:

- 4 (4-ounce / 113-g) boneless, skinless chicken breasts
- 2 tablespoons avocado oil
- 1 cup sliced cremini mushrooms
- 1 cup packed chopped fresh spinach
- 1 pint cherry tomatoes, halved

- ½ cup chopped fresh basil
- ½ red onion, thinly sliced
- 4 garlic cloves, minced
- 2 teaspoons balsamic vinegar

Directions:

⇒ Preheat the oven to 400°F (205°C).

⇒ Arrange the chicken breast in a large baking dish and brush them generously with the avocado oil.

⇒ Mix together the mushrooms, spinach, tomatoes, basil, red onion, cloves, and vinegar in a medium bowl, and toss to combine. Scatter each chicken breast with ¼ of the vegetable mixture.

⇒ Bake in the preheated oven for about 20 minutes, or until the internal temperature reaches at least 165°F (74°C) and juices run clear when pierced with a fork.

⇒ Allow the chicken to rest for 5 to 10 minutes before slicing to serve.

Nutrition: calories: 220 ; fat: 9.1g ; protein: 28.2g ; carbs: 6.9g ; fiber: 2.1g ; sugar: 6.7g ; sodium: 310mg

75)Hidden Valley Chicken Drummies

Preparation Time: **Cooking Time:**   **Servings:6-8**

Ingredients:

- 2 tbsps. Hot sauce
- ½ c. melted butter
- Celery sticks
- 2 packages Hidden Valley dressing dry mix
- 3 tbsps. Vinegar
- 12 chicken drumsticks
- Paprika

Directions:

⇒ Preheat the oven to 350 0F.

⇒ Rinse and pat dry the chicken.

⇒ In a bowl blend the dry dressing, melted butter, vinegar and hot sauce. Stir until combined.

⇒ Place the drumsticks in a large plastic baggie, pour the sauce over drumsticks. Massage the sauce until the drumsticks are coated.

⇒ Place the chicken in a single layer on a baking dish. Sprinkle with paprika.

⇒ Bake for 30 minutes, flipping halfway.

⇒ Serve with crudité or salad.

Nutrition: Calories: 155, Fat:18 g, Carbs:96 g, Protein:15 g, Sugars:0.7 g, Sodium:340 mg

76)Balsamic Chicken And Beans

Preparation Time: **Cooking Time:**   **Servings: 4**

Ingredients:

- 1 lb. trimmed fresh green beans
- ¼ c. balsamic vinegar
- 2 sliced shallots
- 2 tbsps. Red pepper flakes
- 4 skinless, de-boned chicken breasts
- 2 minced garlic cloves
- 3 tbsps. Extra virgin olive oil

Directions:

⇒ Combine 2 tablespoons of the olive oil with the balsamic vinegar, garlic, and shallots. Pour it over the chicken breasts and refrigerate overnight.

⇒ The next day, preheat the oven to 375 0F.

⇒ Take the chicken out of the marinade and arrange in a shallow baking pan. Discard the rest of the marinade.

⇒ Bake in the oven for 40 minutes.

⇒ While the chicken is cooking, bring a large pot of water to a boil.

⇒ Place the green beans in the water and allow them to cook for five minutes and then drain.

⇒ Heat one tablespoon of olive oil in the pot and return the green beans after rinsing them.

⇒ Toss with red pepper flakes.

Nutrition: Calories: 433, Fat:17.4 g, Carbs:12.9 g, Protein:56.1 g, Sugars:13 g, Sodium:292 mg

77)Italian Pork

Preparation Time: **Cooking Time: 1 Hour**   **Servings:6**

Ingredients:

- 2 pounds pork roast
- 3 tablespoons olive oil
- 2 teaspoons oregano, dried
- 1 tablespoon Italian seasoning
- 1 teaspoon rosemary, dried
- 1 teaspoon basil, dried
- 3 garlic cloves, minced
- ¼ cup vegetable stock
- A pinch of salt and black pepper

Directions:

⇒ In a baking pan, combine the pork roast with the oil, the oregano and the other ingredients, toss and bake at 390 degrees F for 1 hour.

⇒ Slice the roast, divide it and the other ingredients between plates and serve.

Nutrition: calories 580, fat 33.6, fiber 0.5, carbs 2.3, protein 64.9

78) Chicken And Brussels Sprouts

Preparation Time: **Cooking Time:**   **Servings:4**

Ingredients:

- 1 cored, peeled and chopped apple
- 1 chopped yellow onion
- 1 tbsp. organic olive oil

- 3 c. shredded Brussels sprouts
- 1 lb. ground chicken meat
- Black pepper

Directions:

⇒ Heat up a pan while using oil over medium-high heat, add chicken, stir and brown for 5 minutes.

⇒ Enjoy!

⇒ Add Brussels sprouts, onion, black pepper and apple, stir, cook for 10 minutes, divide into bowls and serve.

Nutrition: Calories: 200, Fat:8 g, Carbs:13 g, Protein:9 g, Sugars:3.3 g, Sodium:194 mg

79) Chicken Divan

Preparation Time: **Cooking Time:**   **Servings:**

Ingredients:

- 1 c. croutons
- 1 c. cooked and diced broccoli pieces
- ½ c. water

- 1 c. grated extra sharp cheddar cheese
- ½ lb. de-boned and skinless cooked chicken pieces
- 1 can mushroom soup

Directions:

⇒ Preheat the oven to 350°F

⇒ In a large pot, heat the soup and water. Add the chicken, broccoli, and cheese. Combine thoroughly.

⇒ Pour into a greased baking dish.

⇒ Place the croutons over the mixture.

⇒ Bake for 30 minutes or until the casserole is bubbling and the croutons are golden brown.

Nutrition: Calories: 380, Fat:22 g, Carbs:10 g, Protein:25 g, Sugars:2 g, Sodium:475 mg

Chapter 6: Snacks & Desserts Recipes

80) Boiled Cabbage

Preparation Time: **Cooking Time: 5 Minutes**   **Servings:6**

Ingredients:

- 1 large head green cabbage
- 3 cups vegetable broth
- 1 teaspoon salt
- ½ teaspoon black pepper

Directions:

⇒ Place the cabbage, broth, salt, and pepper in the inner pot.
⇒ Cook within 5 minutes. Serve.

Nutrition: Calories 54Fat: 0gProtein: 3gSodium: 321mgFiber: 5gCarbohydrates: 13gSugar: 7g

81) Cereal Mix

Preparation Time: **Cooking Time: 40 Minutes**   **Servings:6**

Ingredients:

- 3 tablespoons extra virgin organic olive oil
- 1 teaspoon hot sauce
- ½ teaspoon garlic powder
- ½ teaspoon onion powder
- ½ teaspoon cumin, ground
- A pinch of red pepper cayenne
- 3 cups rice cereal squares
- 1 cup cornflakes
- ½ cup pepitas

Directions:

⇒ In a bowl, combine the oil while using the hot sauce, garlic powder, onion powder, cumin, cayenne, rice cereal, cornflakes and pepitas.
⇒ Toss and spread on the lined baking sheet.
⇒ Put inside the oven and bake at 350 degrees F for 40 minutes.
⇒ Divide into bowls and serve as a snack.

Nutrition: Calories: 199Fat: 3gFiber: 4gCarbs: 12g Protein: 5g

82) Steamed Broccoli

Preparation Time: **Cooking Time: 1 Minute**   **Servings:6**

Ingredients:

- 6 cups broccoli florets

Directions:

⇒ Pour 1½ cups water into the inner pot of the Instant Pot®. Place a steam rack inside.
⇒ Place the broccoli florets inside a steamer basket and place the basket on the steam rack.
⇒ Steam within 1 minute.
⇒ Remove the steamer basket and serve.

Nutrition: Calories 30Fat: 0gProtein: 3gSodium: 30mgFiber: 2gCarbohydrates: 6gSugar: 2g

83) Berries Cream

Preparation Time: **Cooking Time: 15 Minutes**   **Servings:4**

Ingredients:

- 2 teaspoons lemon juice
- 1-pound blueberries
- 1-pound strawberries

Directions:

⇒ In a small pot, mix the lemon juice with the strawberries and blueberries. Stir, bring to a simmer over medium heat, cook for 15 minutes, divide into bowls and serve cold.
⇒ Enjoy!

Nutrition: calories 132, fat 2, fiber 3, carbs 8, protein 5

84) Turmeric Bars

Preparation Time: **Cooking Time: 10 Minutes**   **Servings:6**

Ingredients:

- 1 cup shredded coconut
- 10 dates, pitted
- 1 tablespoon coconut oil
- 1 teaspoon cinnamon
- 1 ¼ cup coconut butter
- 1 ½ teaspoon turmeric powder
- 2 teaspoons honey
- 1/8 teaspoon black pepper

Directions:

⇒ Prepare a baking pan and line with parchment paper.

⇒ Place the coconut and dates in a food processor and pulse until well-combined. Add in the coconut oil and cinnamon.

⇒ Press the dough at the bottom of the pan and set in the fridge for 2 hours.

⇒ Make the filling by melting the coconut butter in a double boiler. Stir in turmeric powder and honey.

⇒ Pour in the mixture into the pan with the crust.

⇒ Chill within 2 hours.

Nutrition: Calories 410 Total Fat 41g Total Carbs 13g Protein 1g Sugar: 11g Fiber: 2g Sodium: 208mg Potassium 347mg

85) Cinnamon Apple Mix

Preparation Time: **Cooking Time: 20 Minutes**   **Servings:6**

Ingredients:

- 6 apples, cored and roughly chopped
- 4 tablespoons chicory root powder
- 2 teaspoons vanilla extract
- 3 drops lemon oil
- 1 ½ teaspoon ground cinnamon

Directions:

⇒ In a small pot, mix the apples with chicory powder, vanilla, lemon oil and cinnamon. Stir and bring to a simmer over medium heat. Cook for 20 minutes then divide into bowls and serve cold.

⇒ Enjoy!

Nutrition: calories 110, fat 2, fiber 3, carbs 5, protein 5

86) Potato Chips

Preparation Time: **Cooking Time: 30 Minutes**   **Servings:6**

Ingredients:

- 2 gold potatoes, cut into thin rounds
- 1 tablespoon olive oil
- 2 teaspoons garlic, minced

Directions:

⇒ In a bowl, combine the French fries while using the oil along with the garlic, toss, spread more than a lined baking sheet.

⇒ Put inside the oven and bake at 400 degrees F for a half-hour.

⇒ Divide into bowls and serve.

Nutrition: Calories: 200,Fat: 3,Fiber: 5,Carbs: 13,Protein: 6

87) Piquillo Peppers With Cheese

Preparation Time: **Cooking Time: 10 Minutes**   **Servings: 24**

Ingredients:

- 1 canned roasted piquillo peppers
- 2 tbsp olive oil
- 1 tbsp parsley, chopped
- Filling

- 2 oz. goat cheese
- 2 tbsp heavy cream
- 1 tbsp olive oil

Directions:

⇒ Prepare and set up the oven at 370 degrees F.

⇒ Layer a baking tray with some olive oil.

⇒ Whisk all goat cheese with cream and olive oil in a bowl.

⇒ Deseed the peppers and divide the cheese filling into each pepper.

⇒ Place them in the baking tray and drizzle the remaining oil and parsley on top.

⇒ Bake for 10 minutes then serve.

Nutrition: Calories 274 Fat 24.3g, Carbs 4.2g, Protein 11g, Fiber 2g

88) Lemon Garlic Red Chard

Preparation Time: **Cooking Time: 7 Minutes**   **Servings:4**

Ingredients:

- 1 tablespoon avocado oil
- 1 small yellow onion, peeled and diced
- 1 bunch red chard, leaves and stems chopped and kept separate (about 12 ounces)
- 3 cloves garlic, minced

- ¾ teaspoon salt
- Juice from ½ medium lemon
- 1 teaspoon lemon zest

Directions:

⇒ Put the oil to the inner pot and allow it to heat 1 minute. Add the onion and chard stems and sauté 5 minutes. Put the garlic and sauté another 30 seconds. Put the chard leaves, salt, and lemon juice and stir to combine. Turn off. Cook again within 60 seconds.

⇒ Scoop the chard mixture into a serving bowl and top with lemon zest.

Nutrition: Calories 57Fat: 3gProtein: 2gSodium: 617mgFiber: 2gCarbohydrates: 6gSugar: 2g

89) Rice Pudding

Preparation Time: **Cooking Time: 35 Minutes**   **Servings:4**

Ingredients:

- 6 cups almond milk
- Chicory root powder to the taste
- 2 cups black rice, washed and rinsed

- 1 tablespoon ground cinnamon
- ½ cup shredded coconut, unsweetened

Directions:

⇒ In a pot, mix the rice with the milk, chicory powder, cinnamon and coconut. Bring to a simmer over medium-low heat, cook for 35 minutes, divide into bowls to chill then serve cold.

⇒ Enjoy!

Nutrition: calories 170, fat 4, fiber 4, carbs 13, protein 6

90) Lemony Steamed Asparagus

Preparation Time: **Cooking Time: 0 Minutes**   **Servings:4**

Ingredients:

- 1-pound asparagus, woody ends removed
- Juice from ½ large lemon
- ¼ teaspoon kosher salt

Directions:

⇒ Add ½ cup water to the inner pot and add the steam rack. Add the asparagus to the steamer basket and place the basket on top of the rack, then steam within 1 minute.

⇒ Transfer, and top with lemon juice and salt.

Nutrition: Calories 13Fat: 0gProtein: 1gSodium: 146mgFiber: 1gCarbohydrates: 3gSugar: 1g

91) Fresh Veggie Bars

Preparation Time: **Cooking Time: 25 Minutes**   **Servings:18**

Ingredients:

- Egg-1
- Broccoli florets-2 cups
- Cheddar cheese-1/3 cup (grated)
- Onion-¼ cup (peeled and chopped)
- Cauliflower rice-½ cup
- Fresh parsley-2 tablespoons (chopped)
- Olive oil-A drizzle (for greasing)
- Salt and black pepper-to taste (ground)

Directions:

⇒ Warm-up a saucepan with water over medium heat

⇒ Stir into the broccoli and let it simmer for a minute.

⇒ Strain and finely chop it to put it into a bowl.

⇒ Mix in the egg, cheddar cheese, cauliflower rice, salt, pepper, parsley, and mix.

⇒ Give them the shape of bars by using the mixture on your hands.

⇒ Put them on a greased baking sheet.

⇒ Keep it in an oven at 400°F and bake for 20 minutes.

⇒ Settle the prepared dish on a platter to serve.

Nutrition: Calories: 19Fat: 1g Fiber: 3gCarbs: 3gProtein: 3g

92) "cheesy" Brussels Sprouts And Carrots

Preparation Time: **Cooking Time: 10 Minutes**   **Servings:4**

Ingredients:

- 1-pound Brussels sprouts, tough ends removed and cut in half
- 1-pound baby carrots
- 1 cup chicken stock
- 2 tablespoons lemon juice
- ½ cup nutritional yeast
- ¼ teaspoon salt

Directions:

⇒ Add the Brussels sprouts, carrots, stock, lemon juice, nutritional yeast, and salt to the inner pot. Stir well to combine. Cook within 10 minutes.

⇒ Transfer the vegetables and sauce to a bowl and serve.

Nutrition: Calories 134Fat: 1gProtein: 9gSodium: 340mgFiber: 8gCarbohydrates: 23gSugar: 8g

93) Simple Banana Cake

Preparation Time: **Cooking Time: 45 Minutes**   **Servings:4**

Ingredients:

- 1 ½ cups stevia
- 2 cups almond flour
- 3 bananas, peeled and mashed
- 3 eggs

- 2 teaspoon baking powder
- 1 teaspoon ground cinnamon
- 1 teaspoon ground nutmeg

Directions:

⇒ In a bowl, mix the eggs with the stevia, baking powder, cinnamon, nutmeg, banana and flour. Stir well and pour into a greased cake pan then cover with tin foil.

⇒ Place the pan in the oven, bake at 350 degrees F for 45 minutes then let the cake cool, slice and serve.

⇒ Enjoy!

Nutrition: calories 300, fat 11, fiber 11, carbs 12, protein 4

94) Massaged Kale Chips

Preparation Time: **Cooking Time: 20 Minutes**   **Servings:2 cups**

Ingredients:

- 4 cups kale, stemmed, rinsed, drained, torn into 2-inch pieces
- 2 tablespoons extra-virgin olive oil

- 1 teaspoon sea salt
- 2 tablespoons apple cider vinegar

Directions:

⇒ Preheat the oven to 350ºF (180ºC).

⇒ Combine all the ingredients in a large bowl. Stir to mix well.

⇒ Gently massage the kale leaves in the bowl for 5 minutes or until wilted and bright.

⇒ Place the kale on a baking sheet. Bake in the preheated oven for 20 minutes or until crispy. Toss the kale halfway through.

⇒ Remove the kale from the oven and serve immediately.

Nutrition: (1 cup)calories: 138 ; fat: 13.8g ; protein: 1.4g ; carbs: 2.9g ; fiber: 1.2g ; sugar: 0.8g ; sodium: 1176mg

95) Orange And Blackberry Cream

Preparation Time: **Cooking Time: 20 Minutes**   **Servings:6**

Ingredients:

- 5 tablespoons chicory root powder
- 1-ounce orange juice

- 1 pound blackberries

Directions:

⇒ In a pot, mix the blackberries with the orange juice and chicory powder. Stir and bring to a simmer over medium heat.

⇒ Cook for 20 minutes, divide into bowls and serve cold.

⇒ Enjoy!

Nutrition: calories 110, fat 2, fiber 3, carbs 6, protein 6

96) Lemon Ginger Broccoli And Carrots

Preparation Time: **Cooking Time: 5 Minutes**   **Servings:6**

Ingredients:

- 1 tablespoon avocado oil
- 1" fresh ginger, peeled and thinly sliced
- 1 clove garlic, minced
- 2 broccoli crowns, florets

- 2 large carrots, sliced
- ½ teaspoon kosher salt
- Juice from ½ large lemon
- ¼ cup of water

Directions:

⇒ Put the oil to the inner pot. Heat-up within 2 minutes.

⇒ Add the ginger and garlic and sauté 1 minute. Add the broccoli, carrots, and salt and stir to combine. Turn off.

⇒ Add the lemon juice and water and use a wooden spoon to scrape up any brown bits—Cook within 2 minutes.

⇒ Serve immediately.

Nutrition: Calories 67Fat: 2gProtein: 3gSodium: 245mgFiber: 3gCarbohydrates: 10gSugar: 3g

97) Lemony Cauliflower Rice

Preparation Time: **Cooking Time: 8 Minutes**   **Servings:4**

Ingredients:

- 1 tablespoon avocado oil
- 1 small yellow onion, peeled and diced
- 1 teaspoon minced garlic
- 4 cups riced cauliflower

- Juice from 1 little lemon
- ½ teaspoon salt
- ¼ teaspoon black pepper

Directions:

⇒ Put the oil to the pot, and heat 1 minute.

⇒ Add the onion and sauté 5 minutes.

⇒ Add the garlic and sauté 1 more minute.

⇒ Add the cauliflower rice, lemon juice, salt, and pepper and stir to combine—Cook within 1 minute.

⇒ Transfer to a bowl for serving.

Nutrition: Calories 60Fat: 3gProtein: 2gSodium: 311mgFiber: 2gCarbohydrates: 6gSugar: 3g

98) Peppers Avocado Salsa

Preparation Time: **Cooking Time: 12 Minutes**   **Servings:2**

Ingredients:

- 1 and ½ lbs. mixed bell peppers, cut into strips
- 1 tablespoon avocado oil
- ½ cup tomato passata

- 1 avocado, peeled, pitted, and cubed
- Salt and black pepper, to taste

Directions:

⇒ Add bell peppers and all other ingredients to a suitable cooking pot.

⇒ Cover the pot's lid and cook for 12 minutes on medium heat.

⇒ Serve fresh and enjoy.

Nutrition: Calories 304Total Fat 20 g Cholesterol 12 mg Sodium 645 mg Total Carbs 9 g Sugar 2 gFiber 5 g Protein 22 g

99) Cacao Brownies

Preparation Time: **Cooking Time: 3 Hours**   **Servings:4**

Ingredients:

- 3 tablespoons coconut oil, divided
- 1 cup almond butter
- 1 cup unsweetened cacao powder
- ½ cup coconut sugar
- 2 large eggs

- 2 ripe bananas
- 2 teaspoons vanilla extract
- 1 teaspoon baking soda
- ½ teaspoon sea salt

Directions:

⇒ Coat the bottom of the slow cooker with 1 tablespoon of coconut oil.

⇒ In a medium bowl, combine the almond butter, cacao powder, coconut sugar, eggs, bananas, vanilla, baking soda, and salt

⇒ Mash the bananas and stir well until a batter forms

⇒ Pour the batter into the slow cooker.

⇒ Cover the cooker and set to low. Cook for 2½ to 3 hours, until firm to a light touch but still gooey in the middle, and serve.

Nutrition:

Chapter 7: Special Recipes

100) Caesar Dressing

Preparation Time: **Cooking Time: 0 Minutes**   **Servings:2**

Ingredients:

- ¼ Cup Paleo mayonnaise
- 2 Tablespoons Olive Oil
- 2 Cloves Garlic, Minced
- ½ Teaspoon Anchovy Paste

- 1 Tablespoon White Wine Vinegar
- ½ Teaspoon Lemon Zest
- 2 Tablespoons Lemon Juice, Fresh
- Sea Salt & Black Pepper to Taste

Directions:

⇒ Whisk all of your ingredients together. It should be emulsified and combined.

⇒ Put salt and pepper, and then refrigerate it for up to a week.

Nutrition: Calories 167Protein: 0.2 Grams Fat: 18.9 Grams Carbs: 1.3 Grams

101) Massaged Kale And Crispy Chickpea Salad

Preparation Time: **Cooking Time: 15 Minutes**   **Servings:4-6**

Ingredients:

- 1 large bunch kale, rinsed, stemmed, and cut into thin strips
- 2 teaspoons freshly squeezed lemon juice
- 2 tablespoons extra-virgin olive oil, divided
- ¾ teaspoon sea salt, divided

- 1 (14-ounce / 397-g) can cooked chickpeas (about 2 cups)
- 1 teaspoon sweet paprika
- 1 avocado, chopped

Directions:

⇒ Put the kale in a large bowl, then drizzle with 1 tablespoon of olive oil and lemon juice. Sprinkle with ¼ teaspoon of salt.

⇒ Gently knead the kale leaves in the bowl for 5 minutes or until wilted and bright. Rip the leafy part of the kale off the stem, then discard the stem.

⇒ Heat the remaining olive oil in a nonstick skillet over medium-low heat until shimmering.

⇒ Add the chickpeas, paprika, and remaining salt, then cook for 15 minutes or until the chickpeas are crispy.

⇒ Transfer the kale to a large serving bowl, then top with chickpeas and avocado. Toss to combine well and serve.

Nutrition: calories: 359 ; fat: 20.0g ; protein: 13.0g ; carbs: 35.0g ; fiber: 10.0g ; sugars: 1.0g ; sodium: 497mg

102) Garlic Aioli

Preparation Time: **Cooking Time: 0 Minute**   **Servings:4**

Ingredients:

- ½ Cup anti-inflammatory mayonnaise (here)

- 3 garlic cloves, finely minced

Directions:

⇒ In a small bowl, whisk the mayonnaise and garlic to combine.

⇒ Keep refrigerated in a tightly sealed container for up to 4 days.

Nutrition: Calories: 169Total Fat: 20gTotal Carbs: <1gSugar: 0gFiber: 0gProtein: <1gSodium: 36mg

103) Kamut

Preparation Time: **Cooking Time: 15 Minutes**   **Servings:6**

Ingredients:

- 1 cup Kamut berries
- 2 cups water
- 1 teaspoon salt
- 1 onion

- 1 teaspoon turmeric
- 1 teaspoon cilantro
- 1 tablespoon cashew butter

Directions:

⇒ In a large pan, combine the Kamut berries and water together.

⇒ Add salt and close the lid.

⇒ Cook the dish for 50 minutes on the medium heat.

⇒ Meanwhile, peel the onion and chop it into small pieces.

⇒ Combine the chopped onion with the cilantro and turmeric. Stir the mixture.

⇒ Heat a pan and add the cashew butter.

⇒ Add the chopped onion mixture and sauté it for 5 minutes or until the onion is soft.

⇒ When Kamut berries are cooked, remove them from the heat and combine them with the chopped onion mixture.

⇒ Stir it carefully.

⇒ Serve the dish warm.

Nutrition: calories: 149, fat: 0.8g, total carbs: 24.2g, sugars: 0.8g, protein: 4.4g

104) Salmon & Beans Salad

Preparation Time: **Cooking Time: 7 Minutes**   **Servings:4**

Ingredients:

- For Salmon:
- 4 (6-ounce) salmon fillets
- Ground cumin, to taste
- Salt and freshly ground black pepper, to taste
- 2 tablespoons olive oil
- For Salad:
- 1 (15-ounce) can pinto beans, rinsed and drained

- 1 (15-ounce) can kidney beans, rinsed and drained
- 1 (15-ounce) can navy beans, rinsed and drained
- 1 medium bunch scallion, chopped
- 1 small bunch fresh parsley, chopped
- 1/3 cup extra-virgin essential olive oil
- ¼ cup freshly squeezed lemon juice
- Salt and freshly ground black pepper, to taste

Directions:

⇒ Sprinkle the salmon fillets with cumin, salt and black pepper evenly.

⇒ In a sizable nonstick skillet, heat oil on medium heat.

⇒ Ass salmon, skin-side down and cook for about 3-4 minutes.

⇒ Carefully flip the side and cook for about 3 minutes.

⇒ Meanwhile in the bowl, mix together all salad ingredients.

⇒ Top with salmon fillets and serve.

Nutrition: Calories: 429, Fat: 16g, Carbohydrates: 24g, Fiber: 2g, Protein: 40g

105) Spinach Salad With Lemony Dressing

Preparation Time: **Cooking Time: 0 Minutes**   **Servings:4**

Ingredients:

- 2 tablespoons freshly squeezed lemon juice
- ¼ cup Dijon mustard
- 1½ tablespoons maple syrup

- 2 tablespoons extra-virgin olive oil
- ¼ teaspoon sea salt, or to taste
- 6 cups baby spinach leaves

Directions:

⇒ Make the lemon dressing: Combine all the ingredients, except for the spinach, in a small bowl. Stir to mix well.

⇒ Put the spinach in a large serving bowl, the drizzle with the lemon dressing. Toss to combine well. Serve immediately.

Nutrition: calories: 150 ; fat: 14.0g ; protein: 2.0g ; carbs: 8.0g ; fiber: 2.0g ; sugars: 5.0g ; sodium: 362mg

106) Tender Amaranth Cutlets

Preparation Time: **Cooking Time: 15 Minutes**   **Servings:5**

Ingredients:

- 1 cup amaranth, cooked
- 1 teaspoon salt
- 1 egg, whisked
- 2 oz Parmesan
- 1 onion

- 1 tablespoon olive oil
- 1 teaspoon dill
- 1 teaspoon minced garlic
- ½ teaspoon lemon zest

Directions:

⇒ Peel the onion and dice it.

⇒ Heat a skillet and add the olive oil.

⇒ Put the diced onion in the skillet and cook for 5 minutes over medium heat. Stir the mixture frequently.

⇒ In a large bowl, combine the egg, cooked amaranth, onion, minced garlic, salt, and lemon zest.

⇒ Sprinkle the mixture with the dill and stir it carefully until you get a smooth mix.

⇒ Preheat the oven to 350 F.

⇒ Make small balls from the amaranth mixture and flatten them slightly.

⇒ Cover a tray with baking paper and transfer the amaranth balls to the tray.

⇒ Put the tray in the oven and cook the cutlets for 10 minutes.

⇒ When the cutlets are cooked, remove them from the oven and cool them a little.

⇒ Serve the dish immediately.

Nutrition: calories: 276, fat: 6.0g, total carbs: 29.9g, sugars: 1.7g, protein: 21.6g

107) Zoodle Bolognese

Preparation Time: **Cooking Time: 35 Minutes**   **Servings:4**

Ingredients:

- Bolognese
- 3 oz. olive oil
- 1 white onion, chopped
- 1 garlic clove, minced
- 3 oz. celery, chopped
- 3 cups crumbled tofu
- 2 tbsp tomato paste
- 1 ½ cups crushed tomatoes
- 1 tsp salt

- ¼ tsp black pepper
- 1 tbsp dried basil
- 1 tbsp Worcestershire sauce
- Water as needed
- Zoodles
- 2 lbs zucchini
- 2 tbsp butter
- Salt orblack pepper to taste

Directions:

⇒ Pour the olive oil into a saucepan and heat over medium heat. When no longer shimmering, add the onion, garlic, and celery. Sauté for 3 minutes or until the onions are soft and the carrots caramelized.

⇒ Pour in the tofu, tomato paste, tomatoes, salt, black pepper, basil, and Worcestershire sauce. Stir and cook for 15 minutes, or simmer for 30 minutes.

⇒ Mix in some water if the mixture is too thick and simmer further for 20 minutes.

⇒ While the sauce cooks, make the zoodles. Run the zucchini through a spiralizer to form noodles.

⇒ Melt the butter in a skillet over medium heat and toss the zoodles quickly in the butter, about 1 minute only.

⇒ Season with salt and black pepper.

⇒ Divide the zoodles into serving plates and spoon the Bolognese on top. Serve the dish immediately.

Nutrition: Calories:457, Total Fat:37g, Saturated Fat:8.1g, Total Carbs:17g, Dietary Fiber:5g, Sugar:4g, Protein:22g, Sodium:656mg

108) Stir-fry Sauce

Preparation Time: **Cooking Time: 0 Minute**   **Servings:4**

Ingredients:

- ¼ Cup low-sodium soy sauce
- 3 garlic cloves, minced
- Juice of 2 limes
- 1 tablespoon grated fresh ginger
- 1 tablespoon arrowroot powder

Directions:

⇒ In a small bowl, whisk together the soy sauce, garlic, lime juice, ginger, and arrowroot powder.

Nutrition: Calories: 24Total Carbs: 4gSugar: 2gProtein: 1gSodium: 887mg

109) Chicken & Cabbage Salad

Preparation Time: **Cooking Time: 12 Minutes**   **Servings:4**

Ingredients:

- For Chicken Marinade:
- ¼ cup scallion, chopped
- 2 tablespoons fresh ginger, minced
- ¼ cup coconut aminos
- ¼ cup olive oil
- 1 tablespoon honey
- Salt and freshly ground black pepper, to taste
- 2 skinless, boneless chicken breasts
- For Salad:
- ¼ cup balsamic vinegar
- 2 cups red cabbage, shredded
- 1 cup green cabbage, shredded
- 2 cups carrots, peeled and shredded
- 4 cups fresh kale, trimmed and chopped
- 3 scallions, chopped

Directions:

⇒ For chicken in a very bowl, mix together all ingredients except chicken.

⇒ In another bowl, coat chicken with 3 tablespoons of marinade.

⇒ Refrigerate to marinate approximately 30-60 minutes.

⇒ For dressing in a very bowl, mix together remaining marinade and vinegar.

⇒ Preheat the grill to medium-high heat. Grease the grill grate.

⇒ Remove chicken from refrigerator and discard any excess marinade.

⇒ Grill for about 5-6 minutes per side.

⇒ Remove from grill whilst aside to cool down the slightly.

⇒ Cut the chicken breasts in thin slices.

⇒ In a large serving bowl, mix together salad ingredients.

⇒ Add dressing and toss to coat well.

⇒ Top with chicken slices and serve.

Nutrition: Calories: 401, Fat: 6g, Carbohydrates: 29g, Fiber: 14g, Protein: 36g

110) Green Beans With Nuts

Preparation Time: **Cooking Time:**   **Servings:2**

Ingredients:

- 3 minced garlic cloves
- 1 tbsp. olive oil
- ½ c. chopped walnuts
- 2 c. sliced green beans

Directions:

⇒ Boil the beans in salted water until tender.

⇒ Place the beans, garlic and walnuts in a preheated pan and cook for about 5-7 minutes on the stove.

Nutrition: Calories: 285, Fat:24.1 g, Carbs:7.1 g, Protein:10 g, Sugars:3.3 g, Sodium:311 mg

111) Green Beans And Mushroom Sauté

Preparation Time: **Cooking Time: 25 Minutes**   **Servings:6**

Ingredients:

- 1 pound green beans, trimmed
- 8 ounces white mushrooms, sliced
- 1 yellow onion, chopped
- 2 tablespoons olive oil
- ½ cup veggie stock
- A pinch of salt and black pepper

Directions:

⇒ Heat up a big pan with the oil over medium-high heat and add the onion, stir and cook for 4 minutes.

⇒ Add the stock and the mushrooms, then stir and cook for 6 minutes more.

⇒ Add green beans, salt and pepper.

⇒ Toss and cook over medium heat for 15 minutes, then divide everything between plates and serve as a side dish.

Nutrition: Calories 182Fat 4gFiber 5gCarbs 6gProtein 8g

112) Endives And Broccoli

Preparation Time: **Cooking Time: 20 Minutes**   **Servings:4**

Ingredients:

- 2 endives, shredded
- 1 cup broccoli florets
- 2 tablespoons olive oil
- 1 tablespoon walnuts, chopped
- 1 tablespoon almonds, chopped
- 2 garlic cloves, minced
- 1 teaspoon rosemary, dried
- 1 teaspoon cumin, ground
- 1 teaspoon chili powder

Directions:

⇒ In a roasting pan, combine the endives with the broccoli and the other ingredients, toss and bake at 380 degrees F for 20 minutes.

⇒ Divide the mix between plates and serve.

Nutrition: calories 139, fat 9.8, fiber 9.3, carbs 11.9, protein 4.9

113) Beets Stewed With Apples

Preparation Time: **Cooking Time:**   **Servings:2**

Ingredients:

- 2 tbsps. Tomato paste
- 1 tbsps. Olive oil
- 1 c. water
- 2 peeled, cored and sliced apples
- 3 peeled, boiled and grated beets
- 2 tbsps. Sour cream

Directions:

⇒ Boil the beets until half-done

⇒ In a deep pan preheated with olive oil cook the grated beets for 15 minutes.

⇒ Add the sliced apples, tomato paste, sour cream and 1 cup water. Stew for 30 minutes covered.

Nutrition: Calories: 346, Fat:7.7 g, Carbs:26.8 g, Protein:2 g, Sugars:10.2 g, Sodium:96.1 mg

114) Herbed Green Beans

Preparation Time: **Cooking Time:** **Servings:4**

Ingredients:

- ½ c. chopped fresh mint
- 2 minced garlic cloves
- 1 tsp. lemon zest
- 4 c. trimmed green beans

- 1 tbsp. olive oil
- 1 tsp. coarse ground black pepper
- ½ c. chopped fresh parsley

Directions:

⇒ Heat the olive oil in a large sauté pan over medium heat. Add the green beans and garlic.

⇒ Add the mint, parsley, lemon zest, and black pepper. Toss to coat.

⇒ Sauté until the green beans are crisp tender, approximately 5-6 minutes.

⇒ Serve immediately.

Nutrition: Calories: 66.2, Fat:3.5 g, Carbs:8.3 g, Protein:2.1 g, Sugars:2 g, Sodium:65 mg

115) Peanut Sauce

Preparation Time: **Cooking Time: 0 Minute** **Servings:8**

Ingredients:

- 1 cup lite coconut milk
- ¼ cup creamy peanut butter
- ¼ cup freshly squeezed lime juice

- 3 garlic cloves, minced
- 2 tablespoons low-sodium soy sauce, or gluten-free soy sauce, or tamari
- 1 tablespoon grated fresh ginger

Directions:

⇒ In a blender or food processor, process the coconut milk, peanut butter, lime juice, garlic, soy sauce, and ginger until smooth.

⇒ Keep refrigerated in a tightly sealed container for up to 5 days.

Nutrition: Calories: 143Total Fat: 11gTotal Carbs: 8gSugar: 2gFiber: 1gProtein: 6gSodium: 533mg

116) Walnut Pesto

Preparation Time: **Cooking Time: 0 Minute** **Servings:8**

Ingredients:

- ½ Cup walnuts
- ¼ cup extra-virgin olive oil
- 4 garlic cloves, minced

- 1 cup baby spinach
- ¼ cup basil leaves
- ½ teaspoon sea salt

Directions:

⇒ In a blender or food processor, combine the walnuts, olive oil, garlic, spinach, basil, and salt.

⇒ Pulse for 15 to 20 (1-second) bursts, or until everything is finely chopped.

Nutrition: Calories: 106Total Fat: 11gTotal Carbs: 1gSugar: 1gFiber: 1gProtein: 2gSodium: 120mg

117) Mushroom And Cauliflower Rice

Preparation Time: **Cooking Time: 15 Minutes**   **Servings:6**

Ingredients:

- 1½ cups cauliflower rice
- 2 tablespoons olive oil
- 4 ounces wild mushrooms, roughly chopped
- 3 shallots, chopped

- 8 ounces cremini mushrooms, roughly chopped
- 2 cups veggie stock
- A pinch of salt and black pepper
- 2 tablespoons chopped cilantro

Directions:

⇒ Heat up a pot with the oil over medium heat and add the cauliflower rice and shallots.

⇒ Stir and cook for 5 minutes.

⇒ Add stock, cremini mushrooms and wild mushrooms, then stir and cook for 10 minutes more.

⇒ Add the parsley, salt and pepper and mix.

⇒ Divide between plates and serve.

Nutrition: Calories 189Fat 3g - Fiber 4gCarbs 9g - Protein 8g

118) Cabbage Slaw With Cashew Dressing

Preparation Time: **Cooking Time: 0 Minutes**   **Servings:6**

Ingredients:

- Salad:
- 2 carrots, grated
- 1 large head green or red cabbage, sliced thin
- Dressing:
- 1 cup cashews, soaked in water for at least 4 hours, drained

- ¼ cup freshly squeezed lemon juice
- ¾ teaspoon sea salt
- ½ cup water

Directions:

⇒ Combine the carrots and cabbage in a large serving bowl. Toss to combine well.

⇒ Put the ingredients for the dressing in a food processor, then pulse until creamy and smooth.

⇒ Dress the salad, then refrigerate for at least 1 hour before serving.

Nutrition: calories: 208 ; fat: 11.0g ; protein: 7.0g ; carbs: 25.0g ; fiber: 8.0g ; sugars: 4.0g ; sodium: 394mg

119) Basic Brown Rice

Preparation Time: **Cooking Time: 55 Minutes**   **Servings:2**

Ingredients:

- 1 cup of brown rice
- 2½ cups water

- ½ teaspoon salt

Directions:

⇒ Mix the rice, water, plus salt in a medium saucepan. Simmer, uncovered, over medium-high heat.

⇒ Set the heat to low, cover, then simmer within 45 minutes. Do not stir the rice during cooking.

⇒ When no liquid remains, remove the pan from the heat and set it aside to cool for 10 minutes.

⇒ Fluff the rice gently using a fork to avoid sticking.

Nutrition: Calories 138 Total Fat: 1g Saturated Fat: 0g Protein: 3g Total Carbohydrates: 29g Fiber: 1g Sugar: 0g Cholesterol: 0mg

Chapter 8: Anti-Inflammatory Meal Plan for Men

Day 1

1) Carrot Rice With Scrambled Eggs| Calories 230

17) Bean Shawarma Salad| Calories 173

89) Rice Pudding | Calories 170

49) Roast Chicken Dal| Calories 307

102) Garlic Aioli | Calories 169

Day 3

6) Hot Honey Porridge | Calories 172

34) Black Bean Tortilla Wrap | Calories 203

84) Turmeric Bars | Calories 410

65) Balsamic Roast Chicken | Calories 587

107) Zoodle Bolognese | Calories 457

Day 5

15) Power Protein Porridge | Calories 572

28) Brisket With Blue Cheese | Calories 397

87) Piquillo Peppers With Cheese | Calories 274

69) Pork With Thyme Sweet Potatoes | Calories 210

118) Cabbage Slaw With Cashew Dressing | Calories 208

Day 7

7) Breakfast Salad | Calories 188

25) Easy Salmon Salad | Calories 553

90) Lemony Steamed Asparagus | Calories 13

62) Chicken With Broccoli | Calories 300

100) Caesar Dressing | Calories 167

Day 2

5) Gingered Carrot & Coconut Muffins | Calories 352

23) Barbecued Ocean Trout With Garlic And Parsley Dressing | Calories 170

81) Cereal Mix | Calories 199

78) Chicken And Brussels Sprouts | Calories 200

110) Green Beans With Nuts | Calories 285

Day 4

11) Pumpkin & Banana Waffles | Calories 357

40) Leek, Chicken, And Spinach Soup | Calories 256

98) Peppers Avocado Salsa | Calories 304

52) Five-spice Roasted Duck Breasts | Calories 152

115) Peanut Sauce | Calories 143

Day 6

13) Creamy Parmesan Risotto With Mushroom And Cauliflower | Calories 179

37) Valencia Salad | Calories 238

95) Orange And Blackberry Cream | Calories 110

57) Pork With Chili Zucchinis And Tomatoes | Calories 300

114) Herbed Green Beans | Calories 66.2

Chapter 9: Conclusion

I hope this cookbook has allowed you to broaden your vision of all the possibilities you have at your fingertips to have a healthy life and leave behind the discomfort caused by inflammation.

I hope it is the first step in a new lifestyle that will allow you to enjoy your day-to-day life with more planning and significantly improve your quality of life, whether you are an office worker or an athlete, whether you live alone or with your family.

Remember that mealtime is a time to connect with yourself and become aware that what we eat and how we do it really says a lot about us and the way we take care of our body, the only one we will have for life.

If this cookbook has improved your life, remember to share it with your family, friends and colleagues, because sometimes a word is enough to change the lives of those around us for the better.

Keep in mind that if at this moment you do not give yourself the opportunity to start having a healthy diet, later will come the time of illness and negative consequences for your lack of care, so a healthy diet should not be a fad or something momentary but forever.

My most sincere good wishes, and may each recipe that you discovered here be a great experience of life and satisfy your palate.

Anti-Inflammatory Diet Cookbook On A Budget

A Low Cost Meal Plan for Men, for Women and for Families | Delicious and Budget Friendly Recipes for Beginners and Expert to Kickstart your Healthy Lifestyle

By Annette Baker

Chapter 1: Introduction

The anti-inflammatory diet is definitely economical, and will allow you to stay on a budget. But the savings go beyond that, because by preventing inflammation you reduce visits to the doctor or buying anti-inflammatory drugs all the time. You also improve your quality of life, reduce your body and mental stress.

Through this cookbook you will be able to easily plan your budget, enjoy delicious recipes and finally say goodbye to inflammation. Below, I will briefly tell you the main points you should know about the anti-inflammatory diet.

What is the anti-inflammatory diet?

this diet consists of consuming foods that prevent inflammation in a natural way, due to their properties and nutrients. In addition to generating eating habits that improve digestion and reduce inflammation, such as chewing each bite very well, taking the necessary time and walking, at least 10 minutes, after eating.

Why the anti-inflammatory diet saves me money?

One of the main reasons why you will see your household finances improve with the anti-inflammatory diet is because it eliminates the consumption of processed products, sodas and avoids or reduces the consumption of alcohol, which represent an unnecessary and recurrent expense in shopping.

Another reason is that you will save on medical expenses or on medicines and anti-inflammatory treatments, besides, you will be able to plan your food budget because with this cookbook you will have a clear idea of what to buy and in what quantities. Remember that making a shopping list allows you to be on a budget.

What to eat on an anti-inflammatory diet?

The anti-inflammatory diet is based on the intake of fruits, nuts, vegetables, fish, poultry, legumes, tubers, whole grains, seeds, and coconut or olive oil.

Make an anti-inflammatory diet by:

Eliminate partially hydrogenated fatty acids or trans fats.

Fry or season with olive or coconut oil.

Consume natural omega-3 fatty acids from oily fish, algae, seeds and nuts.

Seasoning with turmeric with pepper: turmeric has been shown to reduce inflammation and mixed with pepper promotes intestinal absorption.

Eliminate sugary foods such as sugar, soft drinks, industrial juices and refined flours.

Eat adequate amounts of fiber, present in vegetables, whole grains and nuts. Eating foods rich in magnesium such as green leafy vegetables, legumes, whole grains, nuts, seeds and cocoa.

Chapter 2: Breakfast Recipes

1) Spicy Shakshuka

Preparation Time:	Cooking Time: 37 Minutes	Servings: 4

Ingredients:

- 2-Tbsps extra-virgin olive oil
- 1-bulb onion, minced
- 1 jalapeño, seeded and minced
- 2-cloves garlic, minced
- 1-lb spinach
- Salt and freshly ground black pepper
- ¾-tsp coriander

- 1-tsp dried cumin
- 2-Tbsps harissa paste
- ½-cup vegetable broth
- 8-pcs large eggs
- Red pepper flakes, for serving
- Cilantro, chopped for serving
- Parsley, chopped for serving

Directions:

⇒ Preheat your oven to 350°F.

⇒ Heat the oil in an oven-safe skillet placed over medium heat. Stir in the onion and sauté for 5 minutes.

⇒ Add the jalapeño and garlic, and sauté for a minute, or until fragrant. Add in the spinach, and cook for 5 minutes, or until the leaves entirely wilt.

⇒ Season the mixture with salt and pepper, coriander, cumin, and harissa. Cook further for 1 minute.

⇒ Transfer the mixture to your food processor—puree to a thick consistency. Pour in the broth and puree further until achieving a smooth texture.

⇒ Clean and grease the same skillet with nonstick cooking spray. Pour the pureed mixture. By using a wooden spoon, form eight circular wells.

⇒ Crack each egg gently into the wells. Put the skillet in the oven—Bake for 25 minutes, or poaching the eggs until fully set.

⇒ To serve, sprinkle the shakshuka with red pepper flakes, cilantro, and parsley to taste.

Nutrition: Calories 251Fat: 8.3gProtein: 12.5gSodium: 165mgTotal Carbs: 33.6g

2) 5-minute Golden Milk

Preparation Time:	Cooking Time: 4 Minutes	Servings:1

Ingredients:

- 1 1/2 cups light coconut milk
- 1 1/2 cups unsweetened almond milk
- 1 1/2 tsp ground turmeric
- 1/4 tsp ground ginger

- 1 whole cinnamon stick
- 1 Tbsp coconut oil
- 1 pinch ground black pepper
- Sweetener of choice (i.e., coconut sugar, maple syrup, or stevia to taste)

Directions:

⇒ Add coconut milk, ground turmeric, almond milk, ground ginger, cinnamon stick, coconut oil, black pepper, and preferred sweetener to a small casserole.

⇒ Whisk to mix over medium heat and warm up. Heat to the touch until hot but do not boil-about 4 minutes-whisking regularly.

⇒ Turn off heat and taste to make flavor change. For strong spice + flavor, add more sweetener to taste, or more turmeric or ginger.

⇒ Serve straight away, break between two glasses, and leave the cinnamon stick behind. Best when fresh, although the leftovers can be kept 2-3 days in the refrigerator. Reheat up to temperature on the stovetop or microwave.

Nutrition: Calories 205Fat: 19.5gSodium: 161mgCarbohydrates: 8.9gFiber: 1.1gProtein: 3.2g

3) Breakfast Oatmeal

Preparation Time: **Cooking Time: 8 Minutes**   **Servings: 1**

Ingredients:

- 2/3 cup coconut milk
- 1 egg white, pasture-raised
- ½ cup gluten-free quick-cooking oats
- ½ teaspoon turmeric powder
- ½ teaspoon cinnamon
- ¼ teaspoon ginger

Directions:

⇒ Place the non-dairy milk in a saucepan and heat over medium flame.

⇒ Stir in the egg white and continue whisking until the mixture becomes smooth.

⇒ Add in the rest of the ingredients and cook for another 3 minutes.

Nutrition: Calories 395Total Fat 34gSaturated Fat 7gTotal Carbs 19gNet Carbs 16gProtein 10gSugar: 2gFiber: 3gSodium: 76mgPotassium 459mg

4) No-bake Turmeric Protein Donuts

Preparation Time: **Cooking Time: 0 Minutes**   **Servings: 8**

Ingredients:

- 1 ½ cups raw cashews
- ½ cup medjool dates, pitted
- 1 tablespoon vanilla protein powder
- ½ cup shredded coconut
- 2 tablespoons maple syrup
- ¼ teaspoon vanilla extract
- 1 teaspoon turmeric powder
- ¼ cup dark chocolate

Directions:

⇒ Combine all ingredients except for the chocolate in a food processor.

⇒ Pulse until smooth.

⇒ Roll batter into 8 balls and press into a silicone donut mold.

⇒ Place in the freezer for 30 minutes to set.

⇒ Meanwhile, make the chocolate topping by melting the chocolate in a double boiler.

⇒ Once the donuts have set, remove the donuts from the mold and drizzle with chocolate.

Nutrition: Calories 320Total Fat 26gSaturated Fat 5gTotal Carbs 20gNet Carbs 18gProtein 7gSugar: 9gFiber: 2gSodium: 163 mg Potassium 297mg

5) Cheddar & Kale Frittata

Preparation Time: **Cooking Time:**   **Servings: 6**

Ingredients:

- 1/3 c. sliced scallions
- ¼ tsp. pepper
- 1 diced red pepper
- ¾ c. non-fat milk
- 1 c. shredded sharp low-fat cheddar cheese
- 1 tsp. olive oil
- 5 oz. baby kale and spinach
- 12 eggs

Directions:

⇒ Preheat oven to 375 0F.

⇒ With olive oil, grease a glass casserole dish.

⇒ In a bowl, whisk well all ingredients except for cheese.

⇒ Pour egg mixture in prepared dish and bake for 35 minutes.

⇒ Remove from oven and sprinkle cheese on top and broil for 5 minutes.

⇒ Remove from oven and let it sit for 10 minutes.

⇒ Cut up and enjoy.

Nutrition: Calories: 198, Fat:11.0 g, Carbs:5.7 g, Protein:18.7 g, Sugars:1 g, Sodium:209 mg.

6) Mediterranean Frittata

Preparation Time: **Cooking Time: 20 Minutes**   **Servings:6**

Ingredients:

- Eggs, six
- Feta cheese, crumbled, one quarter cup
- Black pepper, one quarter teaspoon
- Oil, spray, or olive
- Oregano, one teaspoon

- Milk, almond or coconut, one quarter cup
- Sea salt, one teaspoon
- Black olives, chopped, one quarter cup
- Green olives, chopped, one quarter cup
- Tomatoes, diced, one quarter cup

Directions:

⇒ Heat oven to 400. Oil one eight by eight-inch baking dish. Combine the milk into the eggs, and then add other ingredients.

⇒ Pour all of this mixture into the baking dish and bake for twenty minutes.

Nutrition: Calories 107 sugars 2 grams fat 7 grams carb 3 grams protein 7 grams

7) Buckwheat Cinnamon And Ginger Granola

Preparation Time: **Cooking Time: 40 Minutes**   **Servings:5**

Ingredients:

- ¼ cup Chia seeds
- ½ Cup Coconut Flakes
- 1 ½ Cup mixed Raw nuts
- 2 cups of gluten-free oats
- 1 cup of buckwheat groats
- 2 tbsp nut butter
- 4 tbsp of coconut oil

- 1 cup of sunflower seeds
- ½ cup of pumpkin seeds
- 1 ½ - 2 inches piece of ginger
- 1 tsp Ground Cinnamon
- 1/3 cup of Rice Malt Syrup
- 4 tbsp of raw cacao powder – Optional

Directions:

⇒ Preheat the oven up to 180C

⇒ Blitz the nuts in your food processor and quickly blitz to chop roughly. Put the chopped nuts in a bowl and add all the other dry ingredients that combine well–oats, coconut, cinnamon, buckwheat, seeds, and salt in a low heat saucepan, melt the coconut oil gently.

⇒ Add the cacao powder (if used) to the wet mixture and blend. Put the wet batter over the dry mix, then mix well to make sure that everything is coated.

⇒ Move the mixture to a wide baking tray lined with grease-proof paper or coconut oil greased. Be sure to uniformly distribute the mixture for 35-40 minutes, turning the mixture halfway through. Bake until the granola is fresh and golden!

⇒ Serve with your favorite nut milk, coconut yogurt scoop, fresh fruit, and superfoods–goji berries, flax seeds, bee pollen, whatever you like! Mix it up every single day.

Nutrition: Calories 220Carbs: 38gFat: 5gProtein: 7g

8) Cilantro Pancakes

Preparation Time:	Cooking Time: 6-8 Minutes	Servings:6

Ingredients:

- ½ cup tapioca flour
- ½ cup almond flour
- ½ teaspoon chili powder
- ¼ teaspoon ground turmeric
- Salt and freshly ground black pepper, to taste
- 1 cup full- Fat coconut milk
- ½ of red onion, chopped
- 1 (½-inch) fresh ginger piece, grated finely
- 1 Serrano pepper, minced
- ½ cup fresh cilantro, chopped
- Oil, as required

Directions:

⇒ In a big bowl, mix together flours and spices.

⇒ Add coconut milk and mix till well combined.

⇒ Fold within the onion, ginger, Serrano pepper and cilantro.

⇒ Lightly, grease a sizable nonstick skillet with oil and warmth on medium-low heat.

⇒ Add about ¼ cup of mixture and tilt the pan to spread it evenly inside the skillet.

⇒ Cook for around 3-4 minutes from either side.

⇒ Repeat with all the remaining mixture.

⇒ Serve along with your desired topping.

Nutrition: Calories: 331, Fat: 10g, Carbohydrates: 37g, Fiber: 6g, Protein: 28g

9) Raspberry Grapefruit Smoothie

Preparation Time:	Cooking Time: 0 Minutes	Servings:1

Ingredients:

- Juice from 1 grapefruit, freshly squeezed
- 1 banana, peeled and sliced
- 1 cup raspberries

Directions:

⇒ Place all ingredients in a blender and pulse until smooth.

⇒ Chill before serving.

Nutrition: Calories 381Total Fat 0.8gSaturated Fat 0.1gTotal Carbs 96gNet Carbs 85gProtein 4gSugar: 61gFiber: 11gSodium: 11mgPotassium 848mg

10) Turmeric Oven Scrambled Eggs

Preparation Time:	Cooking Time: 15 Minutes	Servings:6

Ingredients:

- 8 to 10 large eggs, pasture-raised
- ½ cup unsweetened almond or coconut milk
- ½ teaspoon turmeric powder
- 1 teaspoon chopped cilantro
- ¼ teaspoon black pepper
- A pinch of salt

Directions:

⇒ Preheat the oven to 3500F.

⇒ Grease a casserole or heat-proof baking dish.

⇒ In a bowl, whisk the egg, milk, turmeric powder, black pepper and salt.

⇒ Pour in the egg mixture into the baking dish.

⇒ Place in the oven and bake for 15 minutes or until the eggs have set.

⇒ Remove from the oven and garnish with chopped cilantro on top.

Nutrition: Calories 203Total Fat 16gSaturated Fat 4gTotal Carbs 5gNet Carbs 4gProtein 10gSugar: 4gFiber: 1gSodium: 303 mg Potassium 321mg

11) Chia And Oat Breakfast Bran

Preparation Time: **Cooking Time:**   **Servings:2**

Ingredients:

- 85 g chopped roasted almonds
- 340 g coconut milk
- 30 g cane sugar
- 2½ g orange zest
- 30 g flax seed mix

- 170 g rolled oats
- 340 g blueberries
- 30 g chia seeds
- 2½ g cinnamon

Directions:

⇒ Add all your wet ingredients together and mix the sugar and milk in with the orange zest.

⇒ Stir in the cinnamon and mix well. Once you are sure the sugar isn't lumpy add in the rolled oats, flax seeds, and chia and then let it sit for a minute.

⇒ Grab two bowls or mason jars and pour the mixture in. Top with the roasted almonds, and store in the fridge.

⇒ Pull it out in the morning and dig in!

Nutrition: Calories: 353, Fat:8 g, Carbs:55 g, Protein:15 g, Sugars:9.9 g, Sodium:96 mg

12) Rhubarb, Apple Plus Ginger Muffin Recipe

Preparation Time: **Cooking Time: 30 Minutes**   **Servings:8**

Ingredients:

- 1/2 teaspoon ground cinnamon
- 1/2 teaspoon ground ginger
- pinch sea salt
- 1/2 cup almond meal (ground almonds)
- 1/4 cup unrefined raw sugar
- 2 tbsp finely chopped crystallized ginger
- 1 tbs ground linseed meal
- 1/2 cup buckwheat flour
- 1/4 cup fine brown rice flour

- 1/4 cup (60ml) olive oil
- 1 large free-range egg
- 1 teaspoon vanilla extract
- 2 tablespoons organic corn flour or true arrowroot
- 2 teaspoons gluten-free baking powder
- 1 cup finely sliced rhubarb
- 1 small apple, peeled and finely diced
- 95ml (1/3 cup + 1 tbsp) rice or almond milk

Directions:

⇒ Pre-heat the oven to 180C/350C. Grease or line 8 1/3 cup (80ml) cup muffin tins with a paper case cap.

⇒ In a medium bowl, put the almond meal, ginger, sugar, and linseed. Sieve over baking powder, flours, and spices and then mix evenly. In the flour mixture, whisk in rhubarb and apple to coat.

⇒ Whisk the milk, sugar, egg, and vanilla in another smaller bowl before pouring into the dry mixture and stirring until combined.

⇒ Divide the batter evenly between tins/paper cases and bake for 20 minutes -25 minutes or until it rises, golden around the edges.

⇒ Remove, then set aside for 5 minutes before transferring onto a wire rack to cool off further.

⇒ Eat warm or at room temperature.

Nutrition: Calories 38Carbs: 9gFat: 0gProtein: 0g

13) Breakfast Grains And Fruits

Preparation Time: **Cooking Time:**   **Servings:6**

Ingredients:

- 1 c. raisins
- ¾ c. quick cooking brown rice
- 1 granny smith apple
- 1 orange

- 8 oz. low fat vanilla yogurt
- 3 c. water
- ¾ c. bulgur
- 1 red delicious apple

Directions:

⇒ On high fire, place a large pot and bring water to a boil.

⇒ Add bulgur and rice. Lower fire to a simmer and cook for ten minutes while covered.

⇒ Turn off fire, set aside for 2 minutes while covered.

⇒ In a baking sheet, transfer and evenly spread grains to cool.

⇒ Meanwhile, peel oranges and cut into sections. Chop and core apples.

⇒ Once grains are cool, transfer to a large serving bowl along with fruits.

⇒ Add yogurt and mix well to coat.

⇒ Serve and enjoy.

Nutrition: Calories: 121, Fat:1 g, Carbs:24.2 g, Protein:3.8 g, Sugars:4.2 g, Sodium:500 mg

14) Perky Paleo Potato & Protein Powder

Preparation Time: **Cooking Time: 0 Minutes**   **Servings:1**

Ingredients:

- 1 small sweet potato, pre-baked and fleshed out
- 1-Tbsp protein powder
- 1 small banana, sliced

- ¼-cup blueberries
- ¼-cup raspberries
- Choice of toppings: cacao nibs, chia seeds, hemp hearts, favorite nut/seed butter (optional)

Directions:

⇒ In a small serving bowl, mash the sweet potato using a fork. Add the protein powder. Mix well until thoroughly combined.

⇒ Arrange the banana slices, blueberries, and raspberries on top of the mixture. Garnish with your desired toppings. You can relish this breakfast meal, either cold or warm.

Nutrition: Calories 302Fat: 10gProtein: 15.3gSodium: 65mgTotal Carbs: 46.7g

15) Tomato Bruschetta With Basil

Preparation Time: **Cooking Time:**   **Servings:8**

Ingredients:

- ½ c. chopped basil
- 2 minced garlic cloves
- 1 tbsp. balsamic vinegar
- 2 tbsps. Olive oil

- ½ tsp. cracked black pepper
- 1 sliced whole wheat baguette
- 8 diced ripe Roma tomatoes
- 1 tsp. sea salt

Directions:

⇒ First, preheat the oven to 375 F.

⇒ In a bowl, dice the tomatoes, mix in balsamic vinegar, chopped basil, garlic, salt, pepper, and olive oil, set aside.

⇒ Slice the baguette into 16-18 slices and for about 10 minutes, place on a baking pan to bake.

⇒ Serve with warm bread slices and enjoy.

⇒ For leftovers, store in an airtight container and put in the fridge. Try putting them over grilled chicken, it is amazing!

Nutrition: Calories: 57, Fat:2.5 g, Carbs:7.9 g, Protein:1.4 g, Sugars:0.2 g, Sodium:261 mg

16) Cinnamon Pancakes With Coconut

Preparation Time: **Cooking Time: 18 Minutes**   **Servings: 2**

Ingredients:

- 2 organic eggs
- 1 tbsp almond flour
- 2oz cream cheese
- ¼ cup shredded coconut and more for garnishing
- ½ tbsp erythritol
- 1/8 tsp salt
- 1 tsp cinnamon
- 4 tbsp stevia
- ½ tbsp olive oil

Directions:

⇒ Crack eggs in a bowl, beat until fluffy and then beat in flour and cream cheese until smooth.

⇒ Add remaining ingredients and then stir until well combined.

⇒ Take a frying pan, place it over medium heat, grease it with oil, then pour in half of the batter and cook for 3 to 4 minutes per side until the pancake has cooked and nicely golden brown.

⇒ Transfer pancake to a plate and cook another pancake in the same manner by using the remaining batter.

⇒ Sprinkle coconut on top of cooked pancakes and serve.

Nutrition: Calories 575, Total Fat 51g, Total Carbs 3.5g, Protein 19g

17) Nutty Blueberry Banana Oatmeal

Preparation Time: **Cooking Time: 2 Hours**   **Servings: 6**

Ingredients:

- 2 cup rolled eats
- 1/4 cup almonds (toasted)
- 1/4 cup walnuts
- 1/4 cup pecans
- 2 tbsp ground flax seeds
- 1 tsp ground ginger
- 1 tsp cinnamon
- 1/4 tsp sea salt
- 2 tbsp coconut sugar
- ½ tsp baking powder
- 2 cups of milk
- 2 bananas
- 1 cup fresh blueberries
- 1 tbsp maple syrup
- 1 tsp vanilla extract
- 1 tbsp melted butter
- Yogurt for serving

Directions:

⇒ In a large bowl, add nuts, flax seeds, baking powder, spices, and coconut sugar and mix.

⇒ In another bowl, beat eggs, milk, maple syrup, and vanilla extract.

⇒ Slice the bananas in half and layer them in the slow cooker pot with blueberries.

⇒ Add oats mixture and pour the milk mixture on the top.

⇒ Drizzle with melted butter,

⇒ Cook the slow cooker on low heat for 4 hours or on high heat for 4 hours. Cook till the liquid is absorbed and oats are golden brown.

⇒ Serve warm and top it off with plain Greek yogurt.

Nutrition: Calories 346 mg Total Fat: 15g Carbohydrates: 45g Protein: 11g Sugar: 17g Fiber 7g Sodium: 145 mg Cholesterol: 39mg

18) Poached Salmon Egg Toast

Preparation Time: **Cooking Time: 4 Minutes**   **Servings: 2**

Ingredients:

- Bread, two slices rye or whole-grain toasted
- Lemon juice, one quarter teaspoon
- Avocado, two tablespoons mashed
- Black pepper, one quarter teaspoon
- Eggs, two poached
- Salmon, smoked, four ounces
- Scallions, one tablespoon sliced thin
- Salt, one eighth teaspoon

Directions:

⇒ Add lemon juice to avocado with pepper and salt. Spread the mixed avocado over the toasted bread slices.

⇒ Lay smoked salmon over toast and top with a poached egg. Top with sliced scallions.

Nutrition: Calories 389 fat 17.2 grams protein 33.5 grams carbs 31.5 grams sugar 1.3 grams fiber 9.3 grams

19) Chia Breakfast Pudding

Preparation Time: **Cooking Time: 0 Minutes**   **Servings: 2**

Ingredients:

- Chia seeds, four tablespoons
- Almond butter, one tablespoon
- Coconut milk, three-fourths cup
- Cinnamon, one teaspoon
- Vanilla, one teaspoon
- Cold coffee, three-fourths cup

Directions:

⇒ Combine all of the fixings well and pour them into a refrigerator-safe container. Cover well and let refrigerate overnight.

Nutrition: Calories 282 carbs 5 grams protein 5.9 grams fat 24 grams

20) Eggs With Cheese

Preparation Time: **Cooking Time:**   **Servings: 1**

Ingredients:

- ¼ c. chopped tomato
- 1 egg white
- 1 chopped green onion
- 2 tbsps. Fat-free milk
- 1 slice whole wheat bread
- 1 egg
- ½ oz. reduced fat grated cheddar cheese

Directions:

⇒ Mix the egg and egg whites in a bowl and add the milk.

⇒ Scramble the mixture in a non-stick frying pan until the eggs cook.

⇒ Meanwhile, toast the bread.

⇒ Spoon the scrambled egg mixture onto the toasted bread and top with the cheese until it melts.

⇒ Add the onion and the tomato.

Nutrition: Calories: 251, Fat:11.0 g, Carbs:22.3 g, Protein:16.9 g, Sugars:1.8 g, Sodium:451 mg

21) Tropical Bowls

Preparation Time: **Cooking Time: 0 Minutes**   **Servings: 2**

Ingredients:

- 1 cup orange juice
- 1 cup mango, peeled and cubed
- 1 cup pineapple, peeled and cubed
- 1 banana, peeled
- 1 teaspoon chia seeds
- A pinch of turmeric powder
- 4 strawberries, sliced

Directions:

⇒ In your blender, mix the orange juice with the mango, pineapple, banana, chia seeds and turmeric

⇒ Pulse well, divide into bowls, top each with the strawberries and serve. Enjoy!

Nutrition: calories 171, fat 3, fiber 6, carbs 8, protein 11

22) Shirataki Pasta With Avocado And Cream

Preparation Time: **Cooking Time: 6 Minutes**   **Servings: 2**

Ingredients:

- ½ packet of shirataki noodles, cooked
- ½ of an avocado
- ½ tsp cracked black pepper
- ½ tsp salt
- ½ tsp dried basil
- 1/8 cup heavy cream

Directions:

⇒ Place a medium pot half full with water over medium heat, bring it to boil, then add noodles and cook for 2 minutes.

⇒ Then drain the noodles and set aside until required.

⇒ Place avocado in a bowl, mash it with a fork,

⇒ Mash avocado in a bowl, transfer it in a blender, add remaining ingredients, and pulse until smooth.

⇒ Take a frying pan, place it over medium heat and when hot, add noodles in it, pour in the avocado mixture, stir well and cook for 2 minutes until hot.

⇒ Serve straight away.

Nutrition: Calories 131, Total Fat 12.6g, Total Carbs 4.9g, Protein 1.2g, Sugar 0.3g, Sodium 588mg

23) Delicious Amaranth Porridge

Preparation Time: **Cooking Time: 30 Minutes**   **Servings: 2**

Ingredients:

- ½ cup water
- 1 cup almond milk, unsweetened
- ½ cup amaranth
- 1 pear, peeled and cubed
- ½ teaspoon ground cinnamon
- ¼ teaspoon fresh ginger, grated
- A pinch of ground nutmeg
- 1 teaspoon maple syrup
- 2 tablespoons chopped pecans

Directions:

⇒ Put the water and the almond milk in a pot, bring to a simmer over medium heat, add the amaranth, mix and cook for 20 minutes.

⇒ Add the pear, cinnamon, ginger, nutmeg and maple syrup and mix. Simmer for 10 minutes more, divide into bowls and serve with pecans sprinkled on top.

⇒ Enjoy!

Nutrition: calories 199, fat 9, fiber 4, carbs 25, protein 3

24) Almond Flour Pancakes With Cream Cheese

Preparation Time: **Cooking Time: 18 Minutes**   **Servings: 2**

Ingredients:

- ½ cup almond flour
- 1 tsp erythritol
- ½ tsp cinnamon
- 2oz cream cheese
- 2 organic eggs
- 1 tbsp unsalted butter

Directions:

⇒ Prepare the pancake batter, and for this, place flour in a blender, add remaining ingredients and pulse for 2 minutes until smooth.

⇒ Tip the batter in a bowl and let it rest for 3 minutes.

⇒ Then take a large skillet pan, place it over medium heat, add butter and when it melts, pour in ¼ of prepared pancake batter.

⇒ Spread the batter evenly in the pan, cook for 2 minutes per side until nicely golden brown and then transfer pancake to a plate.

⇒ Cook three more pancakes in the same manner by using the remaining batter and, when done, serve the pancakes with favorite berries.

Nutrition: Calories 170, Total Fat 14.3g, Total Carbs 4.3, Protein 6.9g, Sugar 0.2g, Sodium 81mg

25) Turkey Apple Breakfast Hash

Preparation Time: **Cooking Time: 10 Minutes**   **Servings:5**

Ingredients:

- For the meat:
- 1 lb. ground turkey
- 1 tablespoon coconut oil
- ½ teaspoon dried thyme
- ½ teaspoon cinnamon
- sea salt, to taste
- For the hash:
- 1 tbsp coconut oil
- 1 onion
- 1 large apple, peeled, cored, and chopped

- 2 cups spinach or greens of choice
- ½ tsp turmeric
- ½ tsp dried thyme
- sea salt, to taste
- 1 large or 2 small zucchinis
- ½ cup shredded carrots
- 2 cups cubed frozen butternut squash (or the sweet potato)
- 1 tsp cinnamon
- ¾ tsp powdered ginger
- ½ tsp garlic powder

Directions:

⇒ In a skillet, heat a spoonful of coconut oil over medium/high heat. Attach turkey to the ground and cook until crispy. Season with thyme, cinnamon, and a pinch of sea salt. Move to the plate.

⇒ Throw remaining coconut oil into the same skillet and sauté onion until softened for 2-3 minutes.

⇒ Add the courgettes, apple, carrots, and frozen squash to taste—Cook for around 4-5 minutes, or until veggies soften.

⇒ Attach and whisk in spinach until wilted.

⇒ Add cooked turkey, seasoning, salt, and shut off oil.

⇒ Enjoy this hash fresh from the pan, or let it cool and refrigerate all week long. The hash can remain in a sealed container in the refrigerator for about 5-6 days.

Nutrition: Calories 350Carbs: 20gFat: 19gProtein: 28g

26) Cheesy Flax And Hemp Seeds Muffins

Preparation Time: **Cooking Time: 30 Minutes**   **Servings:2**

Ingredients:

- 1/8 cup flax seeds meal
- ¼ cup raw hemp seeds
- ¼ cup almond meal
- Salt, to taste
- ¼ tsp baking powder
- 3 organic eggs, beaten

- 1/8 cup nutritional yeast flakes
- ¼ cup cottage cheese, low-fat
- ¼ cup grated parmesan cheese
- ¼ cup scallion, sliced thinly
- 1 tbsp olive oil

Directions:

⇒ Switch on the oven, then set it 360°F and let it preheat.

⇒ Meanwhile, take two ramekins, grease them with oil, and set aside until required.

⇒ Take a medium bowl, add flax seeds, hemp seeds, and almond meal, and then stir in salt and baking powder until mixed.

⇒ Crack eggs in another bowl, add yeast, cottage cheese, and parmesan, stir well until combined, and then stir this mixture into the almond meal mixture until incorporated.

⇒ Fold in scallions, then distribute the mixture between prepared ramekins and bake for 30 minutes until muffins are firm and the top is nicely golden brown.

⇒ When done, take out the muffins from the ramekins and let them cool completely on a wire rack.

⇒ For meal prepping, wrap each muffin with a paper towel and refrigerate for up to thirty-four days.

⇒ When ready to eat, reheat muffins in the microwave until hot and then serve.

Nutrition: Calories 179, Total Fat 10.9g, Total Carbs 6.9g, Protein 15.4g, Sugar 2.3g, Sodium 311mg

Chapter 3: Lunch & Dinner Recipes

27) Chicken And Gluten-free Noodle Soup

Preparation Time: **Cooking Time: 25 Minutes**   **Servings:4**

Ingredients:

- ¼ cup extra-virgin olive oil
- 3 celery stalks, cut into ¼-inch slices
- 2 medium carrots, cut into ¼-inch dice
- 1 small onion, cut into ¼-inch dice
- 1 fresh rosemary sprig
- 4 cups chicken broth

- 8 ounces gluten-free penne
- 1 teaspoon salt
- ¼ teaspoon freshly ground black pepper
- 2 cups diced rotisserie chicken
- ¼ cup finely chopped fresh flat-leaf parsley

Directions:

⇒ Heat-up the oil over high heat in a large pot.

⇒ Put the celery, carrots, onion, and rosemary and sauté until softened, 5 to 7 minutes.

⇒ Add the broth, penne, salt, and pepper and boil.

⇒ Simmer and cook until the penne is tender, 8 to 10 minutes.

⇒ Remove and discard the rosemary sprig, and add the chicken and parsley.

⇒ Reduce the heat to low. Cook within 5 minutes, and serve.

Nutrition: Calories 485 Total Fat: 18g Total Carbohydrates: 47g Sugar: 4g Fiber: 7gProtein: 33gSodium: 1423mg

28) Lentil Curry

Preparation Time: **Cooking Time: 40 Minutes**   **Servings:4**

Ingredients:

- 2 tsp. Mustard Seeds
- 1 tsp. Turmeric, grounded
- 1 cup Lentils, soaked
- 2 tsp. Cumin Seeds
- 1 Tomato, large & chopped
- 1 Yellow Onion, sliced finely
- 4 cups Water

- Sea Salt, as needed
- 2 Carrots, sliced into half-moons
- 3 handful of Spinach leaves, shredded
- 1 tsp. Ginger, minced
- ½ tsp. Chili Powder
- 2 tbsp. Coconut Oil

Directions:

⇒ First, place the mung beans and water in a deep saucepan over medium-high heat.

⇒ Now, bring the beans mixture to a boil and allow it to simmer.

⇒ Simmer within 20 to 30 minutes or until the mung beans are softened.

⇒ Then, heat the coconut oil in a large saucepan over medium heat and stir in the mustard seeds and cumin seeds.

⇒ If the mustard seeds pop, put the onions. Sauté the onions for 4 minutes or until they softened.

⇒ Spoon in the garlic and continue sautéing for another 1 minute. Once aromatic, spoon in the turmeric and chili powder to it.

⇒ Then, add the carrot and tomato—Cook for 6 minutes or until softened.

⇒ Finally, add the cooked lentils to it and give everything a good stir.

⇒ Stir in the spinach leaves and sauté until wilted. Remove from heat. Serve it warm and enjoy.

Nutrition: Calories 290KcalProteins: 14gCarbohydrates: 43gFat: 8g

29) Chicken And Snap Pea Stir-fry

Preparation Time: **Cooking Time: 10 Minutes**   **Servings:4**

Ingredients:

- 1 ¼ cups boneless skinless chicken breast, thinly sliced
- 3 tablespoons fresh cilantro, chopped
- 2 tablespoons vegetable oil
- 2 tablespoons of sesame seeds
- 1 bunch scallions, thinly sliced
- 2 teaspoons Sriracha
- 2 garlic cloves, minced

- 2 tablespoons rice vinegar
- 1 bell pepper, thinly sliced
- 3 tablespoons soy sauce
- 2½ cups snap peas
- Salt, to taste
- Freshly ground black pepper, to taste

Directions:

⇒ Heat-up the oil in a pan over medium heat. Add garlic and thinly sliced scallions. Cook for a minute and then add 2 ½ cups snap peas along with bell pepper. Cook until tender, just for about 3-4 minutes.

⇒ Add chicken and cook for about 4-5 minutes, or until thoroughly cooked.

⇒ Add in 2 teaspoons Sriracha, 2 tablespoons of sesame seeds, 3 tablespoons soy sauce, and 2 tablespoons rice vinegar.

⇒ Toss everything until well-combined. Simmer within 2-3 minutes over low heat.

⇒ Add 3 tablespoons of chopped cilantro and stir well. Transfer, and sprinkle with extra sesame seeds and cilantro, if needed. Enjoy!

Nutrition: 228 calories 11 g fat 11 g total carbs 20 g protein

30) Juicy Broccolini With Anchovy Almonds

Preparation Time: **Cooking Time: 10 Minutes**   **Servings:6**

Ingredients:

- 2 bunches of broccolini, trimmed
- 1 tablespoon extra-virgin olive oil
- 1 long fresh red chili, deseeded, finely chopped
- 2 garlic cloves, thinly sliced

- ¼ cup natural almonds, coarsely chopped
- 2 teaspoons lemon rind, finely grated
- A squeeze of lemon juice, fresh
- 4 anchovies in oil, chopped

Directions:

⇒ Warm the oil until hot in a large saucepan. Add the drained anchovies, garlic, chili, and lemon rind. Cook until aromatic, for 30 seconds, stirring frequently. Add the almond & continue to cook for a minute more, stirring frequently. Remove from the heat & add a squeeze of fresh lemon juice.

⇒ Then place the broccolini in a steamer basket set over a saucepan of simmering water. Cover & cook until crisp-tender, for 2 to 3 minutes. Drain well and then transfer to a large-sized serving plate. Top with the almond mixture. Enjoy.

Nutrition: kcal 350 Fat: 7 g Fiber: 3 g Protein: 6 g

31) Shiitake And Spinach Pattie

Preparation Time: **Cooking Time: 15 Minutes**   **Servings:8**

Ingredients:

- 1 ½ cups shiitake mushrooms, minced
- 1 ½ cups spinach, chopped
- 3 garlic cloves, minced
- 2 onions, minced
- 4 tsp. olive oil
- 1 egg
- 1 ½ cups quinoa, cooked
- 1 ½ tsp. Italian seasoning
- 1/3 cup toasted sunflower seeds, ground
- 1/3 cup Pecorino cheese, grated

Directions:

⇒ Heat olive oil in a saucepan. Once hot, sauté shiitake mushrooms for 3 minutes or until lightly seared. Add in garlic and onion. Sauté for 2 minutes or until fragrant and translucent. Set aside.

⇒ In the same saucepan, heat the remaining olive oil. Add in spinach. Reduce heat, then simmer for 1 minute, drain and transfer to a strainer.

⇒ Chop spinach finely and add into the mushroom mixture. Add egg into the spinach mixture. Fold in cooked quinoa—season with Italian seasoning, then mix until well combined. Sprinkle sunflower seeds and cheese.

⇒ Divide the spinach mixture into patties—Cook patties within 5 minutes or until firm and golden brown. Serve with burger bread.

Nutrition: Calories 43Carbs: 9gFat: 0gProtein: 3g

32) Broccoli Cauliflower Salad

Preparation Time: **Cooking Time: 20 Minutes**   **Servings:6**

Ingredients:

- ¼ tsp. Black Pepper, grounded
- 3 cups Cauliflower Florets
- 1 tbsp. Vinegar
- 1 tsp. Honey
- 8 cups Kale, chopped
- 3 cups Broccoli Florets
- 4 tbsp. Extra Virgin Olive Oil
- ½ tsp. Salt
- 1 ½ tsp. Dijon Mustard
- 1 tsp. Honey
- ½ cup Cherries, dried
- 1/3 cup Pecans, chopped
- 1 cup Manchego cheese, shaved

Directions:

⇒ Preheat the oven to 450 ˚ F and place a baking sheet in the middle rack.

⇒ After that, place cauliflower and broccoli florets in a large bowl.

⇒ To this, spoon in half of the salt, two tablespoons of the oil and pepper. Toss well.

⇒ Now, transfer the mixture to the preheated sheet and bake it for 12 minutes while flipping it once in between.

⇒ Once it becomes tender and golden in color, remove it from the oven and allow it to cool completely.

⇒ In the meantime, mix the remaining two tablespoons of oil, vinegar, honey, mustard, and salt in another bowl.

⇒ Brush this mixture over the kale leaves by messaging the leaves with your hands. Set it aside for 3 to 5 minutes.

⇒ Finally, stir in the roasted vegetables, cheese, cherries, and pecan to the broccoli-cauliflower salad.

Nutrition: Calories: 259KcalProteins: 8.4gCarbohydrates: 23.2gFat: 16.3g

Chapter 4: Fish & Seafood Recipes

33) Broiled White Sea Bass

Preparation Time: **Cooking Time:**   **Servings:2**

Ingredients:

- 1 tsp. minced garlic
- Ground black pepper
- 1 tbsp. lemon juice

- 8 oz. white sea bass fillets
- ¼ tsp. salt-free herbed seasoning blend

Directions:

⇒ Preheat the broiler and position the rack 4 inches from the heat source.

⇒ Lightly spray a baking pan with cooking spray. Place the fillets in the pan. Sprinkle the lemon juice, garlic, herbed seasoning and pepper over the fillets.

⇒ Broil until the fish is opaque throughout when tested with a tip of a knife, about 8 to 10 minutes.

⇒ Serve immediately.

Nutrition: Calories: 114, Fat:2 g, Carbs:2 g, Protein:21 g, Sugars:0.5 g, Sodium:78 mg

34) Baked Tomato Hake

Preparation Time: **Cooking Time:**   **Servings:4-5**

Ingredients:

- ½ c. tomato sauce
- 1 tbsp. olive oil
- Parsley
- 2 sliced tomatoes

- ½ c. grated cheese
- 4 lbs. de-boned and sliced hake fish
- Salt.

Directions:

⇒ Preheat the oven to 400 0F.

⇒ Season the fish with salt.

⇒ In a skillet or saucepan; stir-fry the fish in the olive oil until half-done.

⇒ Take four foil papers to cover the fish.

⇒ Shape the foil to resemble containers; add the tomato sauce into each foil container.

⇒ Add the fish, tomato slices, and top with grated cheese.

⇒ Bake until you get a golden crust, for approximately 20-25 minutes.

⇒ Open the packs and top with parsley.

Nutrition: Calories: 265, Fat:15 g, Carbs:18 g, Protein:22 g, Sugars:0.5 g, Sodium:94.6 mg

35) Seared Haddock With Beets

Preparation Time: **Cooking Time: 30 Minutes**   **Servings:4**

Ingredients:

- 8 beets, peeled and cut into eighths
- 2 shallots, thinly sliced
- 2 tablespoons apple cider vinegar
- 2 tablespoons olive oil, divided

- 1 teaspoon bottled minced garlic
- 1 teaspoon chopped fresh thyme
- Pinch sea salt
- 4 (5-ounce / 142-g) haddock fillets, patted dry

Directions:

⇒ Preheat the oven to 400°F (205°C).

⇒ Combine the beets, shallots, vinegar, 1 tablespoon of olive oil, garlic, thyme, and sea salt in a medium bowl, and toss to coat well. Spread out the beet mixture in a baking dish.

⇒ Roast in the preheated oven for about 30 minutes, turning once or twice with a spatula, or until the beets are tender.

⇒ Meanwhile, heat the remaining 1 tablespoon of olive oil in a large skillet over medium-high heat.

⇒ Add the haddock and sear each side for 4 to 5 minutes, or until the flesh is opaque and it flakes apart easily.

⇒ Transfer the fish to a plate and serve topped with the roasted beets.

Nutrition: calories: 343, fat: 8.8g ; protein: 38.1g ; carbs: 20.9g ; fiber: 4.0g ; sugar: 11.5g; sodium: 540mg

36) Heartfelt Tuna Melt

Preparation Time: **Cooking Time:**   **Servings:4**

Ingredients:

- 3 oz. grated reduced-fat cheddar cheese
- 1/3 c. chopped celery
- Black pepper and salt
- ¼ c. chopped onion

- 2 whole-wheat English muffins
- 6 oz. drained white tuna
- ¼ c. low fat Russian

Directions:

⇒ Preheat broiler. Combine tuna, celery, onion and salad dressing.

⇒ Season with salt and pepper.

⇒ Toast English muffin halves.

⇒ Place split-side-up on baking sheet and top each with 1/4 of tuna mixture.

⇒ Broil 2-3 minutes or until heated through.

⇒ Top with cheese and return to broiler until cheese is melted, about 1 minute longer.

Nutrition: Calories: 320, Fat:16.7 g, Carbs:17.1 g, Protein:25.7 g, Sugars:5.85 g, Sodium:832 mg

37) Lemon Salmon With Kaffir Lime

Preparation Time: **Cooking Time:**   **Servings:8**

Ingredients:

- 1 quartered and bruised lemon grass stalk
- 2 kaffir torn lime leaves
- 1 thinly sliced lemon

- 1 ½ c. fresh coriander leaves
- 1 whole side salmon fillet

Directions:

⇒ Pre-heat the oven to 350∘F.

⇒ Cover a baking pan with foil sheets, overlapping the sides

⇒ Place the Salmon on the foil, top with the lemon, lime leaves, the lemon grass and 1 cup of the coriander leaves. Option: season with salt and pepper.

⇒ Bring the long side of the foil to the center before folding the seal. Roll the ends in order to close up the salmon.

⇒ Bake for 30 minutes.

⇒ Transfer the cooked fish to a platter. Top with fresh coriander. Serve with white or brown rice.

Nutrition: Calories: 103, Fat:11.8 g, Carbs:43.5 g, Protein:18 g, Sugars:0.7 g, Sodium:322 mg

Chapter 5: Meat Recipes

38) Peach Chicken Treat

Preparation Time: **Cooking Time:**   **Servings: 4-5**

Ingredients:

- 2 minced garlic cloves
- ¼ c. balsamic vinegar
- 4 sliced peaches
- 4 skinless, deboned chicken breasts

- ¼ c. chopped basil
- 1 tbsp. olive oil
- 1 chopped shallot
- ¼ tsp. black pepper

Directions:

⇒ Heat up the oil in a saucepan over medium-high flame.

⇒ Add the meat and season with black pepper; fry for 8 minutes on each side and set aside to rest in a plate.

⇒ In the same pan, add the shallot and garlic; stir and cook for 2 minutes.

⇒ Add the peaches; stir and cook for 4-5 more minutes.

⇒ Add the vinegar, cooked chicken, and basil; toss and simmer covered for 3-4 minutes more.

⇒ Serve warm.

Nutrition: Calories: 270, Fat:0 g, Carbs:6.6 g, Protein:1.5 g, Sugars:24 g, Sodium:87 mg

39) Ground Pork Pan

Preparation Time: **Cooking Time: 15 Minutes**   **Servings:4**

Ingredients:

- 2 garlic cloves, minced
- 2 red chilies, chopped
- 2 tablespoons olive oil
- 2 pounds pork stew meat, ground
- 1 red bell pepper, chopped
- 1 green bell pepper, chopped

- 1 tomato, cubed
- ½ cup mushrooms, halved
- A pinch of sea salt and black pepper
- 1 tablespoon basil, chopped
- 2 tablespoons coconut aminos

Directions:

⇒ Heat up a pan with the oil over medium heat, add the garlic, chilies, bell peppers, tomato and the mushrooms and sauté for 5 minutes.

⇒ Add the meat and the rest of the ingredients, toss, cook over medium heat for 10 minutes more, divide between plates and serve.

Nutrition: calories 200, fat 3, fiber 5, carbs 7, protein 17

40) Parsley Pork And Artichokes

Preparation Time: **Cooking Time: 35 Minutes**   **Servings:4**

Ingredients:

- 2 tablespoons balsamic vinegar
- 1 cup canned artichoke hearts, drained and quartered
- 2 tablespoons olive oil
- 2 pounds pork stew meat, cubed
- 2 tablespoons parsley, chopped

- 1 teaspoon cumin, ground
- 1 teaspoon turmeric powder
- 2 garlic cloves, minced
- A pinch of sea salt and black pepper

Directions:

⇒ Heat up a pan with the oil over medium heat, add the meat and brown for 5 minutes.

⇒ Add the artichokes, the vinegar and the other ingredients, toss, cook over medium heat for 30 minutes, divide between plates and serve.

Nutrition: calories 260, fat 5, fiber 4, carbs 11, protein 20

41) Pork With Thyme Sweet Potatoes

Preparation Time: **Cooking Time: 35 Minutes**   **Servings:4**

Ingredients:

- 2 sweet potatoes, peeled and cut into wedges
- 4 pork chops
- 3 spring onions, chopped
- 1 tablespoon thyme, chopped
- 2 tablespoons olive oil

- 4 garlic cloves, minced
- A pinch of sea salt and black pepper
- ½ cup vegetable stock
- ½ tablespoon chives, chopped

Directions:

⇒ In a roasting pan, combine the pork chops with the potatoes and the other ingredients, toss gently and cook at 390 degrees F for 35 minutes.

⇒ Divide everything between plates and serve.

Nutrition: calories 210, fat 12.2, fiber 5.2, carbs 12, protein 10

42) Curry Pork Mix

Preparation Time: **Cooking Time: 30 Minutes**   **Servings:4**

Ingredients:

- 2 tablespoon olive oil
- 4 scallions, chopped
- 2 garlic cloves, minced
- 2 pounds pork stew meat, cubed
- 2 tablespoons red curry paste

- 1 teaspoon chili paste
- 2 tablespoons balsamic vinegar
- ¼ cup vegetable stock
- ¼ cup parsley, chopped

Directions:

⇒ Heat up a pan with the oil over medium-high heat, add the scallions and the garlic and sauté for 5 minutes.

⇒ Add the meat and brown for 5 minutes more.

⇒ Add the remaining ingredients, toss, cook over medium heat for 20 minutes, divide between plates and serve.

Nutrition: calories 220, fat 3, fiber 4, carbs 7, protein 12

43) Stir-fried Chicken And Broccoli

Preparation Time: **Cooking Time: 10 Minutes**   **Servings:4**

Ingredients:

- 3 tablespoons extra-virgin olive oil
- 1½ cups broccoli florets
- 1½ pounds (680 g) boneless, skinless chicken breasts, cut into bite-size pieces
- ½ onion, chopped

- ½ teaspoon sea salt
- ⅛ teaspoon freshly ground black pepper
- 3 garlic cloves, minced
- 2 cups cooked brown rice

Directions:

⇒ Heat the olive oil in a large nonstick skillet over medium-high heat until shimmering.

⇒ Add the broccoli, chicken, and onion to the skillet and stir well. Season with sea salt and black pepper.

⇒ Stir-fry for about 8 minutes, or until the chicken is golden browned and cooked through.

⇒ Toss in the garlic and cook for 30 seconds, stirring constantly, or until the garlic is fragrant.

⇒ Remove from the heat to a plate and serve over the cooked brown rice.

Nutrition: calories: 344 ; fat: 14.1g ; protein: 14.1g ; carbs: 40.9g ; fiber: 3.2g ; sugar: 1.2g ; sodium: 275mg

44) Chicken And Broccoli

Preparation Time: **Cooking Time:**   **Servings:4**

Ingredients:

- 2 minced garlic cloves
- 4 de-boned, skinless chicken breasts
- ½ c. coconut cream
- 1 tbsp. chopped oregano

- 2 c. broccoli florets
- 1 tbsp. organic olive oil
- 1 c. chopped red onions

Directions:

⇒ Heat up a pan while using the oil over medium-high heat, add chicken breasts and cook for 5 minutes on each side.

⇒ Add onions and garlic, stir and cook for 5 minutes more.

⇒ Add oregano, broccoli and cream, toss everything, cook for ten minutes more, divide between plates and serve.

⇒ Enjoy!

Nutrition: Calories: 287, Fat:10 g, Carbs:14 g, Protein:19 g, Sugars:10 g, Sodium:1106 mg

45) Pork With Cabbage And Kale

Preparation Time: **Cooking Time: 35 Minutes**   **Servings:4**

Ingredients:

- 1-pound pork stew meat, cut into strips
- 2 tablespoons olive oil
- 1 yellow onion, chopped
- A pinch of sea salt and black pepper
- cup green cabbage, shredded

- ½ cup baby kale
- 2 tablespoons oregano, dried
- 2 tablespoons balsamic vinegar
- ¼ cup vegetable stock

Directions:

⇒ Heat up a pan with the oil over medium-high heat, add the onion and the meat and brown for 5 minutes.

⇒ Add the cabbage and the other ingredients, toss gently and bake everything at 390 degrees F for 30 minutes.

⇒ Divide the whole mix between plates and serve.

Nutrition: calories 331, fat 18.7, fiber 2.1, carbs 6.5, protein 34.2

46) Mediterranean Chicken Bake With Vegetables

Preparation Time: **Cooking Time: 20 Minutes**   **Servings:4**

Ingredients:

- 4 (4-ounce / 113-g) boneless, skinless chicken breasts
- 2 tablespoons avocado oil
- 1 cup sliced cremini mushrooms
- 1 cup packed chopped fresh spinach
- 1 pint cherry tomatoes, halved

- ½ cup chopped fresh basil
- ½ red onion, thinly sliced
- 4 garlic cloves, minced
- 2 teaspoons balsamic vinegar

Directions:

⇒ Preheat the oven to 400°F (205°C).

⇒ Arrange the chicken breast in a large baking dish and brush them generously with the avocado oil.

⇒ Mix together the mushrooms, spinach, tomatoes, basil, red onion, cloves, and vinegar in a medium bowl, and toss to combine. Scatter each chicken breast with ¼ of the vegetable mixture.

⇒ Bake in the preheated oven for about 20 minutes, or until the internal temperature reaches at least 165°F (74°C) and juices run clear when pierced with a fork.

⇒ Allow the chicken to rest for 5 to 10 minutes before slicing to serve.

Nutrition: calories: 220 ; fat: 9.1g ; protein: 28.2g ; carbs: 6.9g ; fiber: 2.1g ; sugar: 6.7g ; sodium: 310mg

47) Hidden Valley Chicken Drummies

Preparation Time:	Cooking Time:	Servings: 6-8

Ingredients:

- 2 tbsps. Hot sauce
- ½ c. melted butter
- Celery sticks
- 2 packages Hidden Valley dressing dry mix
- 3 tbsps. Vinegar
- 12 chicken drumsticks
- Paprika

Directions:

⇒ Preheat the oven to 350 0F.

⇒ Rinse and pat dry the chicken.

⇒ In a bowl blend the dry dressing, melted butter, vinegar and hot sauce. Stir until combined.

⇒ Place the drumsticks in a large plastic baggie, pour the sauce over drumsticks. Massage the sauce until the drumsticks are coated.

⇒ Place the chicken in a single layer on a baking dish. Sprinkle with paprika.

⇒ Bake for 30 minutes, flipping halfway.

⇒ Serve with crudité or salad.

Nutrition: Calories: 155, Fat:18 g, Carbs:96 g, Protein:15 g, Sugars:0.7 g, Sodium:340 mg

48) Balsamic Chicken And Beans

Preparation Time:	Cooking Time:	Servings: 4

Ingredients:

- 1 lb. trimmed fresh green beans
- ¼ c. balsamic vinegar
- 2 sliced shallots
- 2 tbsps. Red pepper flakes
- 4 skinless, de-boned chicken breasts
- 2 minced garlic cloves
- 3 tbsps. Extra virgin olive oil

Directions:

⇒ Combine 2 tablespoons of the olive oil with the balsamic vinegar, garlic, and shallots. Pour it over the chicken breasts and refrigerate overnight.

⇒ The next day, preheat the oven to 375 0F.

⇒ Take the chicken out of the marinade and arrange in a shallow baking pan. Discard the rest of the marinade.

⇒ Bake in the oven for 40 minutes.

⇒ While the chicken is cooking, bring a large pot of water to a boil.

⇒ Place the green beans in the water and allow them to cook for five minutes and then drain.

⇒ Heat one tablespoon of olive oil in the pot and return the green beans after rinsing them.

⇒ Toss with red pepper flakes.

Nutrition: Calories: 433, Fat:17.4 g, Carbs:12.9 g, Protein:56.1 g, Sugars:13 g, Sodium:292 mg

49) Italian Pork

Preparation Time:	Cooking Time: 1 Hour	Servings: 6

Ingredients:

- 2 pounds pork roast
- 3 tablespoons olive oil
- 2 teaspoons oregano, dried
- 1 tablespoon Italian seasoning
- 1 teaspoon rosemary, dried
- 1 teaspoon basil, dried
- 3 garlic cloves, minced
- ¼ cup vegetable stock
- A pinch of salt and black pepper

Directions:

⇒ In a baking pan, combine the pork roast with the oil, the oregano and the other ingredients, toss and bake at 390 degrees F for 1 hour.

⇒ Slice the roast, divide it and the other ingredients between plates and serve.

Nutrition: calories 580, fat 33.6, fiber 0.5, carbs 2.3, protein 64.9

50) Chicken And Brussels Sprouts

Preparation Time: **Cooking Time:**   **Servings:4**

Ingredients:

- 1 cored, peeled and chopped apple
- 1 chopped yellow onion
- 1 tbsp. organic olive oil

- 3 c. shredded Brussels sprouts
- 1 lb. ground chicken meat
- Black pepper

Directions:

⇒ Heat up a pan while using oil over medium-high heat, add chicken, stir and brown for 5 minutes.

⇒ Add Brussels sprouts, onion, black pepper and apple, stir, cook for 10 minutes, divide into bowls and serve.

⇒ Enjoy!

Nutrition: Calories: 200, Fat:8 g, Carbs:13 g, Protein:9 g, Sugars:3.3 g, Sodium:194 mg

51) Chicken Divan

Preparation Time: **Cooking Time:**   **Servings:**

Ingredients:

- 1 c. croutons
- 1 c. cooked and diced broccoli pieces
- ½ c. water

- 1 c. grated extra sharp cheddar cheese
- ½ lb. de-boned and skinless cooked chicken pieces
- 1 can mushroom soup

Directions:

⇒ Preheat the oven to 350°F

⇒ In a large pot, heat the soup and water. Add the chicken, broccoli, and cheese. Combine thoroughly.

⇒ Pour into a greased baking dish.

⇒ Place the croutons over the mixture.

⇒ Bake for 30 minutes or until the casserole is bubbling and the croutons are golden brown.

Nutrition: Calories: 380, Fat:22 g, Carbs:10 g, Protein:25 g, Sugars:2 g, Sodium:475 mg

52) Sumptuous Indian Chicken Curry

Preparation Time: **Cooking Time: 20 Minutes**   **Servings:6**

Ingredients:

- 2 tablespoons coconut oil, divided
- 2 (4-ounce / 113-g) boneless, skinless chicken breasts, cut into bite-size pieces
- 2 medium carrots, diced
- 1 small white onion, diced
- 1 tablespoon minced fresh ginger
- 6 garlic cloves, minced
- 1 cup sugar snap peas, diced
- 1 (5.4-ounce / 153-g) can unsweetened coconut cream

- 1 tablespoon sugar-free fish sauce
- 1 cup low-sodium chicken broth
- ½ cup diced tomatoes, with juice
- 1 tablespoon curry powder
- ¼ teaspoon sea salt
- Pinch cayenne pepper, to taste
- Freshly ground black pepper, to taste
- ¼ cup filtered water

Directions:

⇒ Heat 1 tablespoon of coconut oil in a nonstick skillet over medium-high heat until melted.

⇒ Add the chicken breasts to the skillet and cook for 15 minutes or until an instant-read thermometer inserted in the thickest part of the chicken breasts registers at least 165°F (74°C). Flip the chicken breasts halfway through the cooking time.

⇒ Meanwhile, in a separate skillet, heat the remaining coconut oil over medium heat until melted.

⇒ Add the carrots, onion, ginger, and garlic to the skillet and sauté for 5 minutes or until fragrant and the onion is translucent.

⇒ Add the peas, coconut cream, fish sauce, chicken broth, tomatoes, curry powder, salt, cayenne pepper, black pepper, and water to the skillet. Stir to mix well.

⇒ Bring to a boil. Reduce the heat to medium-low then simmer for 10 minutes.

⇒ Add the cooked chicken to the second skillet, then cook for 2 more minutes to combine well.

⇒ Pour the curry on a large serving plate, then serve immediately.

Nutrition: calories: 223 ; fat: 15.7g ; protein: 13.4g ; carbs: 9.4g ; fiber: 3.0g ; sugar: 2.3g ; sodium: 673mg

53) Pork With Balsamic Onion Sauce

Preparation Time: **Cooking Time: 35 Minutes**   **Servings:4**

Ingredients:

- 1 yellow onion, chopped
- 4 scallions, chopped
- 2 tablespoons avocado oil
- 1 tablespoon rosemary, chopped
- 1 tablespoon lemon zest, grated

- 2 pounds pork roast, sliced
- 2 tablespoons balsamic vinegar
- ½ cup vegetable stock
- A pinch of sea salt and black pepper

Directions:

⇒ Heat up a pan with the oil over medium heat, add the onion and the scallions and sauté for 5 minutes.

⇒ Add the rest of the ingredients except the meat, stir, and simmer for 5 minutes.

⇒ Add the meat, toss gently, cook over medium heat for 25 minutes, divide between plates and serve.

Nutrition: calories 217, fat 11, fiber 1, carbs 6, protein 14

54) Pork With Pears And Ginger

Preparation Time: **Cooking Time: 35 Minutes**   **Servings:4**

Ingredients:

- 2 green onions, chopped
- 2 tablespoons avocado oil
- 2 pounds pork roast, sliced
- ½ cup coconut aminos

- 1 tablespoon ginger, minced
- 2 pears, cored and cut into wedges
- ¼ cup vegetable stock
- 1 tablespoon chives, chopped

Directions:

⇒ Heat up a pan with the oil over medium heat, add the onions and the meat and brown for 2 minutes on each side.

⇒ Add the rest of the ingredients, toss gently and bake at 390 degrees F for 30 minutes.

⇒ Divide the mix between plates and serve.

Nutrition: calories 220, fat 13.3, fiber 2, carbs 16.5, protein 8

55) Butter Chicken

Preparation Time: **Cooking Time:**   **Servings:6**

Ingredients:

- 8 finely chopped garlic cloves
- ¼ c. chopped low-fat unsalted butter
- Freshly ground black pepper

- 6 oz. skinless, de-boned chicken thighs
- 1 tsp. lemon pepper

Directions:

⇒ In a large slow cooker, place chicken thighs.

⇒ Top chicken thighs with butter evenly.

⇒ Sprinkle with garlic, lemon pepper and black pepper evenly.

⇒ Set the slow cooker on low.

⇒ Cover and cook for about 6 hours.

Nutrition: Calories: 438, Fat:28 g, Carbs:14 g, Protein:30 g, Sugars:2 g, Sodium:700 mg

56) Hot Chicken Wings

Preparation Time: | **Cooking Time:** | **Servings:4-5**

Ingredients:

- 2 tbsps. Honey
- ½ stick margarine
- 2 tbsps. Cayenne pepper

- 1 bottle durkee hot sauce
- 10 - 20 chicken wings
- 10 shakes Tabasco sauce

Directions:

⇒ In a deep pot, heat the canola oil. Deep-fry the wings until cooked, approximately 20 minutes.

⇒ In a medium bowl, mix the hot sauce, honey, tabasco, and cayenne pepper. Mix well.

⇒ Place the cooked wings on paper towels. Drain the excess oil.

⇒ Toss the chicken wings in the sauce until coated evenly.

Nutrition: Calories: 102, Fat:14 g, Carbs:55 g, Protein:23 g, Sugars:0.3 g, Sodium:340 mg

57) Chicken, Pasta And Snow Peas

Preparation Time: | **Cooking Time:** | **Servings:1-2**

Ingredients:

- Fresh ground pepper
- 2 ½ c. penne pasta
- 1 standard jar tomato and basil pasta sauce

- 1 c. halved and trimmed snow peas
- 1 lb. chicken breasts
- 1 tsp. olive oil

Directions:

⇒ In a medium frying pan, heat the olive oil. Season the chicken breasts with salt and pepper. Cook the chicken breasts until cooked through for approximately 5 – 7 minutes each side.

⇒ Cook the pasta according to instructions on package. Cook the snow peas with the pasta.

⇒ Scoop 1 cup of the pasta water. Drain the pasta and peas, set aside.

⇒ Once the chicken is cooked, slice diagonally.

⇒ Add the chicken back to the frying pan. Add the pasta sauce. If the mixture seems dry.

⇒ Add some of the pasta water to desired consistency. Heat together.

⇒ Divide into bowls and serve immediately.

Nutrition: Calories: 140, Fat:17 g, Carbs:52 g, Protein:34 g, Sugars:2.3 g, Sodium:400 mg

58) Apricot Chicken Wings

Preparation Time: | **Cooking Time:** | **Servings:3-4**

Ingredients:

- 1 medium jar apricot preserve
- 1 package Lipton onion dry soup mix

- 1 medium bottle Russian dressing
- 2 lbs. chicken wings

Directions:

⇒ Pre-heat the oven to 350∘F.

⇒ Rinse and pat dry the chicken wings.

⇒ Place the chicken wings on a baking pan, single layer.

⇒ Bake for 45 – 60 minutes, turning halfway.

⇒ In a medium bowl, combine the Lipton soup mix, apricot preserve and Russian dressing.

⇒ Once the wings are cooked, toss with the sauce, until the pieces are coated.

⇒ Serve immediately with a side dish.

Nutrition: Calories: 162, Fat:17 g, Carbs:76 g, Protein:13 g, Sugars:24 g, Sodium:700 mg

59) Champion Chicken Pockets

Preparation Time: **Cooking Time:**   **Servings:4**

Ingredients:

- ½ c. chopped broccoli
- 2 halved whole wheat pita bread rounds
- ¼ c. bottled reduced-fat ranch salad dressing
- ¼ c. chopped pecans or walnuts

- 1 ½ c. chopped cooked chicken
- ¼ c. plain low-fat yogurt
- ¼ c. shredded carrot

Directions:

⇒ In a small bowl stir together yogurt and ranch salad dressing.

⇒ In a medium bowl combine chicken, broccoli, carrot, and, if desired, nuts. Pour yogurt mixture over chicken; toss to coat.

⇒ Spoon chicken mixture into pita halves.

Nutrition: Calories: 384, Fat:11.4 g, Carbs:7.4 g, Protein:59.3 g, Sugars:1.3 g, Sodium:368.7 mg

60) Stovetop Barbecued Chicken Bites

Preparation Time: **Cooking Time:**   **Servings:4**

Ingredients:

- 1 diced medium bell pepper
- 1 tbsp. canola oil
- 1 c. tangy, spicy, and sweet barbecue sauce
- Freshly ground black pepper

- 1 diced medium onion
- 1 lb. de-boned skinless chicken breasts
- 3 minced garlic cloves

Directions:

⇒ Wash chicken breasts and pat dry. Cut into bite-sized chunks.

⇒ Heat oil in a large sauté pan over medium heat. Add chicken, onion, garlic, and bell pepper, and cook, stirring, for 5 minutes.

⇒ Add the barbecue sauce and stir to combine. Reduce heat to medium-low and cover pan. Cook, stirring frequently, until chicken is fully cooked, about 15 minutes.

⇒ Remove from heat. Season to taste with freshly ground black pepper and serve immediately.

Nutrition: Calories: 191, Fat:5 g, Carbs:8 g, Protein:27 g, Sugars:0 g, Sodium:480 mg

61) Chicken And Radish Mix

Preparation Time: **Cooking Time:**   **Servings:4**

Ingredients:

- 10 halved radishes
- 1 tbsp. organic olive oil
- 2 tbsps. Chopped chives

- 1 c. low-sodium chicken stock
- 4 chicken things
- Black pepper

Directions:

⇒ Heat up a pan with all the oil over medium-high heat, add chicken, season with black pepper and brown for 6 minutes on either side.

⇒ Add stock and radishes, reduce heat to medium and simmer for twenty minutes.

⇒ Add the chives, toss, divide between plates and serve.

⇒ Enjoy!

Nutrition: Calories: 247, Fat:10 g, Carbs:12 g, Protein:22 g, Sugars:1.1 g, Sodium:673 mg

62) Chicken And Sweet Potato Stew

Preparation Time: **Cooking Time: 40 Minutes**   **Servings:4**

Ingredients:

- 1 tablespoon extra virgin olive oil
- 2 garlic cloves, sliced
- 1 white onion, chopped
- 14 ounces (397 g) tomatoes, chopped
- 2 tablespoons chopped rosemary leaves

- Sea salt and ground black pepper, to taste
- 4 free-range skinless chicken thighs
- 4 sweet potatoes, peeled and cubed
- 2 tablespoons basil leaves

Directions:

⇒ Preheat the oven to 375°F (190°C).

⇒ Heat the olive oil in a nonstick skillet over medium heat until shimmering.

⇒ Add the garlic and onion to the skillet and sauté for 5 minutes or until fragrant and the onion is translucent.

⇒ Add the tomatoes, rosemary, salt, and ground black pepper and cook for 15 minutes or until lightly thickened.

⇒ Arrange the chicken thighs and sweet potatoes on a baking sheet, then pour the mixture in the skillet over the chicken and sweet potatoes. Stir to coat well. Pour in enough water to make sure the liquid cover the chicken and sweet potatoes.

⇒ Bake in the preheated oven for 20 minutes or until the internal temperature of the chicken reaches at least 165°F (74°C).

⇒ Remove the baking sheet from the oven and pour them in a large bowl. Sprinkle with basil and serve.

Nutrition: calories: 297 ; fat: 8.7g ; protein: 22.2g ; carbs: 33.1g ; fiber: 6.5g ; sugar: 9.3g; sodium: 532mg

63) Rosemary Beef Ribs

Preparation Time: **Cooking Time: 2 Hours**   **Servings:4**

Ingredients:

- 1½ pounds (680 g) boneless beef short ribs
- ½ teaspoon garlic powder
- 1 teaspoon salt
- ½ teaspoon freshly ground black pepper

- 2 tablespoons olive oil
- 2 cups low-sodium beef broth
- 1 cup red wine
- 4 sprigs rosemary

Directions:

⇒ Preheat the oven to 350°F (180°C).

⇒ On a clean work surface, rub the short ribs with garlic powder, salt, and black pepper. Let stand for 10 minutes.

⇒ Heat the olive oil in an oven-safe skillet over medium-high heat.

⇒ Add the short ribs and sear for 5 minutes or until well browned. Flip the ribs halfway through. Transfer the ribs onto a plate and set aside.

⇒ Pour the beef broth and red wine into the skillet. Stir to combine well and bring to a boil. Turn down the heat to low and simmer for 10 minutes until the mixture reduces to two thirds.

⇒ Put the ribs back to the skillet. Add the rosemary sprigs. Put the skillet lid on, then braise in the preheated oven for 2 hours until the internal temperature of the ribs reads 165°F (74°C).

⇒ Transfer the ribs to a large plate. Discard the rosemary sprigs. Pour the cooking liquid over and serve warm.

Nutrition: calories: 731 ; fat: 69.1g ; carbs: 2.1g ; fiber: 0g ; protein: 25.1g ; sodium: 781mg

64) Chicken, Bell Pepper & Spinach Frittata

Preparation Time: **Cooking Time:**   **Servings:8**

Ingredients:

- ¾ c. frozen chopped spinach
- ¼ tsp. garlic powder
- ¼ c. chopped red onion
- 1 1/3 c. finely chopped cooked chicken

- 8 eggs
- Freshly ground black pepper
- 1½ c. chopped and seeded red bell pepper

Directions:

⇒ Grease a large slow cooker.

⇒ In a bowl, add eggs, garlic powder and black pepper and beat well.

⇒ Place remaining ingredients into prepared slow cooker.

⇒ Pour egg mixture over chicken mixture and gently, stir to combine.

⇒ Cover and cook for about 2-3 hours.

Nutrition: Calories: 250.9, Fat:16.3 g, Carbs:10.8 g, Protein:16.2 g, Sugars:4 g, Sodium:486 mg

65) Roast Chicken Dal

Preparation Time: **Cooking Time:**   **Servings:4**

Ingredients:

- 15 oz. rinsed lentils
- ¼ c. low-fat plain yogurt
- 1 minced small onion
- 4 c. de-boned, skinless and roasted chicken

- 2 tsps. Curry powder
- 1 ½ tsps. Canola oil
- 14 oz. fire-roasted diced tomatoes
- ¼ tsp. salt

Directions:

⇒ Heat oil in a large heavy saucepan over medium-high heat.

⇒ Add onion and cook, stirring, until softened but not browned, 3 to 4 minutes.

⇒ Add curry powder and cook, stirring, until combined with the onion and intensely aromatic, 20 to 30 seconds.

⇒ Stir in lentils, tomatoes, chicken and salt and cook, stirring often, until heated through.

⇒ Remove from the heat and stir in yogurt. Serve immediately.

Nutrition: Calories: 307, Fat:6 g, Carbs:30 g, Protein:35 g, Sugars:0.1 g, Sodium:361 mg

66) Oregano Pork

Preparation Time: **Cooking Time: 8 Hours**   **Servings:4**

Ingredients:

- 2 pounds pork roast, sliced
- 2 tablespoons oregano, chopped
- ¼ cup balsamic vinegar
- 1 cup tomato paste
- 1 tablespoon sweet paprika

- 1 teaspoon onion powder
- 2 tablespoons chili powder
- 2 garlic cloves, minced
- A pinch of salt and black pepper

Directions:

⇒ In your slow cooker, combine the roast with the oregano, the vinegar and the other ingredients, toss, put the lid on and cook on Low for 8 hours.

⇒ Divide everything between plates and serve.

Nutrition: calories 300, fat 5, fiber 2, carbs 12, protein 24

67) Chicken And Avocado Bake

Preparation Time: **Cooking Time:**   **Servings:4**

Ingredients:

- 2 thinly sliced green onion stalks
- Mashed avocado
- 170 g non-fat Greek yogurt

- 1 ¼ g salt
- 4 chicken breasts
- 15 g blackened seasoning

Directions:

⇒ Start by putting your chicken breast in a plastic zip lock bag with the blackened seasoning. Close and shake, then marinate for about 2-5 minutes.

⇒ As your chicken is marinating, go ahead and put your Greek Yogurt, mashed avocado, and salt in your blender and pulse until smooth.

⇒ Place a large skillet or cast-iron pan on the stove at medium heat, oil the pan and cook the chicken until it is cooked through. You'll need about 5 minutes on each side. However, try not to dry the juices and plate it as soon as the meat is cooked.

⇒ Top with the yogurt mixture.

Nutrition: Calories: 296, Fat:13.5 g, Carbs:6.6 g, Protein:35.37 g, Sugars:0.8 g, Sodium:173 mg

68) Five-spice Roasted Duck Breasts

Preparation Time: **Cooking Time:**   **Servings:4**

Ingredients:

- 1 tsp. five-spice powder
- ¼ tsp. cornstarch
- 2 orange juice and zest
- 1 tbsp. reduced-sodium soy sauce

- 2 lbs. de-boned duck breast
- ½ tsp. kosher salt
- 2 tsps. Honey

Directions:

⇒ Preheat oven to 375 0F.

⇒ Place duck skin-side down on a cutting board. Trim off all excess skin that hangs over the sides. Turnover and make three parallel, diagonal cuts in the skin of each breast, cutting through the fat but not into the meat. Sprinkle both sides with five-spice powder and salt.

⇒ Place the duck skin-side down in an ovenproof skillet over medium-low heat.

⇒ Cook until the fat is melted and the skin is golden brown, about 10 minutes. Transfer the duck to a plate; pour off all the fat from the pan. Return the duck to the pan skin-side up and transfer to the oven.

⇒ Roast the duck for 10 to 15 minutes for medium, depending on the size of the breast, until a thermometer inserted into the thickest part registers 150 0F.

⇒ Transfer to a cutting board; let rest for 5 minutes.

⇒ Pour off any fat remaining in the pan (take care, the handle will still be hot); place the pan over medium-high heat and add orange juice and honey. Bring to a simmer, stirring to scrape up any browned bits.

⇒ Add orange zest and soy sauce and continue to cook until the sauce is slightly reduced, about 1 minute. Stir cornstarch mixture then whisk into the sauce; cook, stirring, until slightly thickened, 1 minute.

⇒ Remove the duck skin and thinly slice the breast meat. Drizzle with the orange sauce.

Nutrition: Calories: 152, Fat:2 g, Carbs:8 g, Protein:24 g, Sugars:5 g, Sodium:309 mg

69) Pork Chops With Tomato Salsa

Preparation Time: **Cooking Time: 15 Minutes**   **Servings:4**

Ingredients:

- 4 pork chops
- 1 tablespoon olive oil
- 4 scallions, chopped
- 1 teaspoon cumin, ground
- ½ tablespoon hot paprika
- 1 teaspoon garlic powder
- A pinch of sea salt and black pepper

- 1 small red onion, chopped
- 2 tomatoes, cubed
- 2 tablespoons lime juice
- 1 jalapeno, chopped
- ¼ cup cilantro, chopped
- 1 tablespoon lime juice

Directions:

⇒ Heat up a pan with the oil over medium heat, add the scallions and sauté for 5 minutes.

⇒ Add the meat, cumin paprika, garlic powder, salt and pepper, toss, cook for 5 minutes on each side and divide between plates.

⇒ In a bowl, combine the tomatoes with the remaining ingredients, toss, divide next to the pork chops and serve.

Nutrition: calories 313, fat 23.7, fiber 1.7, carbs 5.9, protein 19.2

70) Tuscan Chicken With Tomatoes, Olives, And Zucchini

Preparation Time: **Cooking Time: 20 Minutes**   **Servings:4**

Ingredients:

- 4 boneless, skinless chicken breast halves, pounded to ½- to ¾-inch thickness
- 1 teaspoon garlic powder
- ½ teaspoon sea salt
- ⅛ teaspoon freshly ground black pepper
- 2 tablespoons extra-virgin olive oil

- 2 cups cherry tomatoes
- ½ cup sliced green olives
- 1 zucchini, chopped
- ¼ cup dry white wine

Directions:

⇒ On a clean work surface, rub the chicken breasts with garlic powder, salt, and ground black pepper.

⇒ Heat the olive oil in a nonstick skillet over medium-high heat until shimmering.

⇒ Add the chicken and cook for 16 minutes or until the internal temperature reaches at least 165°F (74°C). Flip the chicken halfway through the cooking time. Transfer to a large plate and cover with aluminum foil to keep warm.

⇒ Add the tomatoes, olives, and zucchini to the skillet and sauté for 4 minutes or until the vegetables are soft.

⇒ Add the white wine to the skillet and simmer for 1 minutes.

⇒ Remove the aluminum foil and top the chicken with the vegetables and their juices, then serve warm.

Nutrition: calories: 172 ; fat: 11.1g ; protein: 8.2g ; carbs: 7.9g ; fiber: 2.1g ; sugar: 4.2g ; sodium: 742mg

71) Pork Salad

Preparation Time: **Cooking Time: 10 Minutes**   **Servings:4**

Ingredients:

- 1-pound pork stew meat, cut into strips
- 3 tablespoons olive oil
- 4 scallions, chopped
- 2 tablespoons lemon juice
- 2 tablespoons balsamic vinegar

- 2 cups mixed salad greens
- 1 avocado, peeled, pitted and roughly cubed
- 1 cucumber, sliced
- 2 tomatoes, cubed
- A pinch of salt and black pepper

Directions:

⇒ Heat up a pan with 2 tablespoons of oil over medium heat, add the scallions, the meat and the lemon juice, toss and cook for 10 minutes.

⇒ In a salad bowl, combine the salad greens with the meat and the remaining ingredients, toss and serve.

Nutrition: calories 225, fat 6.4, fiber 4, carbs 8, protein 11

72) Lime Pork And Green Beans

Preparation Time: **Cooking Time: 40 Minutes**   **Servings:4**

Ingredients:

- 2 pounds pork stew meat, cubed
- 2 tablespoons avocado oil
- ½ cup green beans, trimmed and halved
- 2 tablespoons lime juice

- 1 cup coconut milk
- 1 tablespoon rosemary, chopped
- A pinch of salt and black pepper

Directions:

⇒ Heat up a pan with the oil over medium heat, add the meat and brown for 5 minutes.

⇒ Add the rest of the ingredients, toss gently, bring to a simmer and cook over medium heat for 35 minutes more.

⇒ Divide the mix between plates and serve.

Nutrition: calories 260, fat 5, fiber 8, carbs 9, protein 13

73) Pork With Chili Zucchinis And Tomatoes

Preparation Time: **Cooking Time: 35 Minutes**   **Servings:4**

Ingredients:

- 2 tomatoes, cubed
- 2 pounds pork stew meat, cubed
- 4 scallions, chopped
- 2 tablespoons olive oil
- 1 zucchini, sliced

- Juice of 1 lime
- 2 tablespoons chili powder
- ½ tablespoons cumin powder
- A pinch of sea salt and black pepper

Directions:

⇒ Heat up a pan with the oil over medium heat, add the scallions and sauté for 5 minutes.

⇒ Add the meat and brown for 5 minutes more.

⇒ Add the tomatoes and the other ingredients, toss, cook over medium heat for 25 minutes more, divide between plates and serve.

Nutrition: calories 300, fat 5, fiber 2, carbs 12, protein 14

74) Pork With Olives

Preparation Time: **Cooking Time: 40 Minutes**   **Servings:4**

Ingredients:

- 1 yellow onion, chopped
- 4 pork chops
- 2 tablespoons olive oil
- 1 tablespoon sweet paprika

- 2 tablespoons balsamic vinegar
- ¼ cup kalamata olives, pitted and chopped
- 1 tablespoon cilantro, chopped
- A pinch of sea salt and black pepper

Directions:

⇒ Heat up a pan with the oil over medium heat, add the onion and sauté for 5 minutes.

⇒ Add the meat and brown for 5 minutes more.

⇒ Add the rest of the ingredients, toss, cook over medium heat for 30 minutes, divide between plates and serve.

Nutrition: calories 280, fat 11, fiber 6, carbs 10, protein 21

75) Green Enchiladas Chicken Soup

Preparation Time: **Cooking Time: 6 Hours**   **Servings: 12**

Ingredients:

- 2½ lbs. chicken thighs or breasts, skinless or boneless
- 24 oz. chicken broth
- 28 oz. green enchilada sauce
- 1 oz. green salsa
- 1 oz. cubed cream cheese, room temp
- Monterey Jack cheese
- Pepper and salt to taste

Directions:

⇒ Place chicken, chicken broth, and green enchilada sauce into a slow cooker.

⇒ Cook for about 6-8 hours on low. Remove the chicken and shred it.

⇒ Scoop 1-2 ladles soup into a bowl then stir in half and half. Place back into the slow cooker.

⇒ Add shredded chicken, green salsa, cream cheese, and jack cheese. Turn your slow cooker to warm, then stir for cheeses to melt.

⇒ Add more salsa or hot sauce to taste.

⇒ Top with topping of choice i.e. cilantro, avocado, sour cream, or green onion.

Nutrition: Calories: 328Fats: 19.7gCarbs: 6gProtein: 30.8gSugars: 2.8gFiber: 0.5gSodium: 690mgPotassium: 528mg

Chapter 6: Snacks & Dessert Recipes

76) Olives Parsley Spread

| Preparation Time: | Cooking Time: 10 Minutes | Servings:4 |

Ingredients:

- 2 cups black olives, pitted and halved
- 2 garlic cloves, minced
- 1 tablespoon lemon juice
- 1 tablespoon olive oil
- ¼ cup chicken stock
- Salt and black pepper, to taste

Directions:

⇒ Add black olive, chicken stock, and all other ingredients to a suitable cooking pot.

⇒ Cover the pot's lid and cook for 10 minutes on medium heat.

⇒ Blend this mixture using a handheld blender.

⇒ Serve fresh and enjoy.

Nutrition: Calories 124 Total Fat 13.4 g Cholesterol 20 mg Sodium 136 mg Total Carbs 6.4 g Sugar 2.1 g Fiber 4.8 g Protein 4.2 g

77) Spinach Cabbage Slaw

| Preparation Time: | Cooking Time: 2 Minutes | Servings:2 |

Ingredients:

- 2 cups red cabbage, shredded
- 1 tablespoon mayonnaise
- 1 spring onion, chopped
- 1-lb. baby spinach
- ½ cup chicken stock

Directions:

⇒ Start by adding onion to a suitable pan, to sauté for 2 minutes.

⇒ Add spinach, stock and mayonnaise then mix well.

⇒ Serve fresh and enjoy.

Nutrition: Calories 194 Total Fat 21.7 g Saturated Fat 9.4 g Total Carbs 8.3 g Sugar 1.6 g Fiber 1.3 g Protein 3.2 g

78) Glazed Pears With Hazelnuts

| Preparation Time: | Cooking Time: 15 Minutes | Servings:4 |

Ingredients:

- 4 pears, peeled, cored, and quartered lengthwise
- 1 cup apple juice
- 1 tablespoon grated fresh ginger
- ½ cup pure maple syrup
- ¼ cup chopped hazelnuts

Directions:

⇒ Put the pears in a large pot, then pour the apple juice over. Bring to a boil over medium-high heat.

⇒ Reduce the heat to medium-low, then cover and simmer for 15 minutes or until the pears are tender.

⇒ Meanwhile, put the ginger and maple syrup in a saucepan. Bring to a boil over medium-high heat. Stir constantly. Turn off the heat and let stand until ready to use.

⇒ Transfer the simmered pears onto a large plate, then glaze with the gingered maple syrup. Spread the hazelnuts on top and serve warm.

Nutrition: calories: 285 ; fat: 2.9g ; protein: 2.1g ; carbs: 66.8g ; fiber: 7.2g ; sugar: 50.2g ; sodium: 9mg

79) Passion Fruit Cream

Preparation Time: **Cooking Time: 50 Minutes**   **Servings:6**

Ingredients:

- 1 cup lemon curd
- 4 passion fruits, pulp and seeds
- 3 ½ ounces maple syrup
- 3 eggs

- 2 ounces coconut oil, melted
- 3 ½ ounces almond milk
- ½ cup almond flour
- ½ teaspoon baking powder

Directions:

⇒ In a bowl, mix the lemon curd with passion fruit, maple syrup, eggs, coconut oil, milk, flour and baking powder. Stir well and divide into 6 cups. Put the cups in an oven pan, fill the pan halfway with water and place in the oven at 200 degrees F.

⇒ Bake for 50 minutes, cool them down and serve.

⇒ Enjoy!

Nutrition: calories 220, fat 12, fiber 3, carbs 7, protein 8

80) Broccoli With Parsley Butter

Preparation Time: **Cooking Time: 8 Minutes**   **Servings:24**

Ingredients:

- 2 tbsp parsley, chopped
- 1 head broccoli, cut into florets

- Salt and black pepper to taste
- ¼ cup butter

Directions:

⇒ Place broccoli in boiling water for 3 minutes then drain.

⇒ Put a suitable pan over moderate heat and add butter to melt.

⇒ Toss in the broccoli, salt, black pepper and parsley.

⇒ Stir and cook for 5 minutes then serve.

Nutrition: Calories 105 Fat 7.5g, Carbs 5.1g, Protein 4g, Fiber 1.1g

81) Butternut Squash Fries

Preparation Time: **Cooking Time: 40 Minutes**   **Servings:4**

Ingredients:

- 1 large butternut squash, peeled, deseeded, and cut into fry-size pieces, about 3 inches long and ½ inch thick
- 2 tablespoons coconut oil

- ¾ teaspoon sea salt
- 3 fresh rosemary sprigs, stemmed and chopped (about 1½ tablespoons)

Directions:

⇒ Preheat the oven to 375°F (190°C). Line a baking sheet with parchment paper.

⇒ Put the butternut squash in a large bowl, then drizzle with coconut oil and sprinkle with salt. Toss to coat well.

⇒ Arrange the butternut squash pieces in the single layer on the prepared baking sheet.

⇒ Bake in the preheated oven for 40 minutes or until golden brown and crunchy. Flip the zucchini fries at least three times during the cooking and top the fries with rosemary sprigs halfway through.

⇒ Transfer the fries on a cooling rack and allow to cool for a few minutes. Serve warm.

Nutrition: calories: 191 ; fat: 6.8g ; protein: 3.0g ; carbs: 34.1g ; fiber: 7.2g ; sugar: 5.9g ; sodium: 451mg

82) Warm Cinnamon-turmeric Almond Milk

Preparation Time:

Cooking Time: 4 Hours

Servings:4

Ingredients:

- 4 cups unsweetened almond milk
- 4 cinnamon sticks
- 2 tablespoons coconut oil
- 1 (4-inch) piece turmeric root, roughly chopped
- 1 (2-inch) piece fresh ginger, roughly chopped
- 1 teaspoon raw honey, plus more to taste

Directions:

⇒ In your slow cooker, combine the almond milk, cinnamon sticks, coconut oil, turmeric, and ginger.

⇒ Cover the cooker and set to low. Cook for 3 to 4 hours.

⇒ Pour the contents of the cooker through a fine-mesh sieve into a clean container; discard the solids.

⇒ Starting with just 1 teaspoon, add raw honey to taste.

Nutrition: Calories: 133Total Fat: 11gTotal Carbs: 10gSugar: 7gFiber: 1g Protein: 1g Sodium: 152mg

83) White Fish Ceviche With Avocado

Preparation Time:

Cooking Time: 0 Minutes

Servings:6

Ingredients:

- Juice of 5 limes
- Juice of 8 lemons
- 1 pound (454 g) fresh wild white fish, cut into ½-inch cubes
- 1 teaspoon minced fresh ginger
- 3 cloves garlic, minced
- 1 cup minced red onions
- ½ cup minced fresh cilantro
- 1 teaspoon Himalayan salt
- 1 teaspoon ground black pepper
- ½ medium Hass avocado, peeled, pitted, and diced

Directions:

⇒ Combine the lime juice and lemon juice in a large bowl, then dunk the fish cubes in the mixture, press so the fish is submerged in the juice.

⇒ Cover the bowl in plastic and refrigerate for at least 40 minutes.

⇒ Meanwhile, combine the ginger, garlic, onions, cilantro, salt, and ground black pepper in a small bowl.

⇒ Stir to mix well.

⇒ Remove the fish bowl from the refrigerator, then sprinkle with the powder mixture. Toss to coat well.

⇒ Spread the diced avocado over the ceviche and serve immediately.

Nutrition: calories: 159 ; fat: 4.9g ; protein: 19.0g ; carbs: 11.6g ; fiber: 2.0g ; sugar: 3.2g ; sodium: 677mg

84) Mango And Nigella Seeds Stew

Preparation Time:

Cooking Time: 20 Minutes

Servings:8

Ingredients:

- 1 ½ pounds mango, peeled and cubed
- 1 teaspoon nigella seeds
- ½ cup apple cider vinegar
- 1 inch ginger, grated
- 1 tablespoon ground cinnamon
- 4 cloves

Directions:

⇒ In a small pot, combine the mango with the nigella seeds, vinegar, ginger, cinnamon and cloves. Stir, bring to a boil over medium-high heat and cook for 20 minutes.

⇒ Divide into bowls and serve cold.

⇒ Enjoy!

Nutrition: calories 140, fat 2, fiber 2, carbs 8, protein 9

85) Vanilla Turmeric Orange Juice

Preparation Time: **Cooking Time: 0 Minutes**   **Servings:2**

Ingredients:

- 3 oranges, peeled and quartered
- 1 cup almond milk, unsweetened
- 1 teaspoon vanilla extract
- ½ teaspoon cinnamon
- ¼ teaspoon turmeric
- a pinch of pepper

Directions:

⇒ Place all ingredients in a blender. Pulse until smooth.

⇒ Put into glasses, then chill in the fridge before serving.

Nutrition: Calories 188 Total Fat 5g Total Carbs 33g Protein 5g Sugar 27g Fiber: 6g Sodium: 53mg

86) Cauliflower Hummus

Preparation Time: **Cooking Time: 0 Minutes**   **Servings:4**

Ingredients:

- 1 medium head cauliflower, trimmed and chopped
- 2 garlic cloves, chopped
- 2 tablespoons of almond butter
- 2 tablespoons olive oil
- 1/8 teaspoon ground cumin
- Salt, to taste
- Pinch of cayenne pepper

Directions:

⇒ In a large pan with boiling water, add cauliflower and cook for about 4-5 minutes.

⇒ Remove from heat and drain well. Keep aside to cool it slightly.

⇒ In a food processor, add cauliflower, butter, cumin, and salt and pulse till smooth.

⇒ Transfer into a serving bowl. Sprinkle with cayenne pepper and serve immediately.

Nutrition: Calories 213Total Fat 8.5 g Saturated Fat 3.1 g Cholesterol 120 mg Sodium 497 mg Total Carbs 21.4 g Fiber 0 g Sugar 0 g Protein 0.1g

87) Cinnamon Pecans

Preparation Time: **Cooking Time: 4 Hours**   **Servings: 3 ½ Cups**

Ingredients:

- 1 tablespoon coconut oil
- 1 large egg white
- 2 tablespoons ground cinnamon
- 2 teaspoons vanilla extract
- ¼ cup maple syrup
- 2 tablespoons coconut sugar
- ¼ teaspoon sea salt
- 3 cups pecan halves

Directions:

⇒ Coat the slow cooker with the coconut oil.

⇒ In a medium bowl, whisk the egg white.

⇒ Add the cinnamon, vanilla, maple syrup, coconut sugar, and salt. Whisk well to combine.

⇒ Add the pecans and stir to coat. Pour the pecans into the slow cooker.

⇒ Cover the cooker and set to low. Cook for 3 to 4 hours.

⇒ Remove the pecans from the slow cooker and spread them on a baking sheet or another cooling surface.

⇒ Let cool for 5 to 10 minutes before serving.

⇒ Store in an airtight container at room temperature for up to 2 weeks.

Nutrition: Calories: 195Total Fat: 18gTotal Carbs: 9gSugar: 6gFiber: 3gProtein: 2gSodium: 46mg

88) Frozen Blueberry Yogurt Bites

Preparation Time:	Cooking Time: 0 Minutes	Servings: 50 Bites

Ingredients:

- 2 cups plain whole-milk yogurt
- 1 banana

- ½ cup fresh blueberries
- 1 tablespoon raw honey

Directions:

⇒ Line a baking sheet with a piece of wax paper.

⇒ Pulse the banana, yogurt, blueberries, and honey in a blender until smooth and creamy.

⇒ Transfer the smooth mixture to a large resealable plastic bag with the corner snipped off. Squeeze the mixture into quarter-sized dots onto the prepared baking sheet. Transfer to the freezer to freeze until solid.

⇒ Store leftovers in an airtight container in the freezer.

Nutrition: (8 bites)calories: 91 ; fat: 3.1g ; protein: 3.0g ; carbs: 12.8g ; fiber: 1.0g ; sugar: 10.0g ; sodium: 29mg

Chapter 7: Special Recipes

89) Braised Bok Choy With Mushrooms

Preparation Time: **Cooking Time: 5 To 10 Minutes**   **Servings:4**

Ingredients:

- 1 tablespoon coconut oil
- 8 baby bok choy, halved lengthwise
- 1 cup shiitake mushrooms, stemmed and thinly sliced
- ½ cup water
- 1 tablespoon coconut aminos
- Sea salt and freshly ground black pepper, to taste
- 1 scallion, sliced thin
- 1 tablespoon toasted sesame seeds

Directions:

⇒ Melt the coconut oil in a large skillet over high heat.

⇒ Add the bok choy, mushrooms, water, and coconut aminos to the skillet. Braise the vegetables for about 5 to 10 minutes, covered, or until the bok choy is softened.

⇒ Remove from the heat and sprinkle the salt and pepper to season.

⇒ Divide the bok choy and mushrooms among plates. Scatter each plate evenly with the scallions and sesame seeds. Serve immediately.

Nutrition: calories: 286 ; fat: 8.2g ; protein: 25.9g ; carbs: 43.1g ; fiber: 18.0g ; sugar: 21.2g ; sodium: 1184mg

90) White Pizza With Mixed Mushrooms

Preparation Time: **Cooking Time: 25 Minutes**   **Servings:4**

Ingredients:

- Crust:
- 2 tbsp flax egg + 6 tbsp water
- ½ cup vegan mayonnaise
- ¾ cup almond flour
- 1 tbsp psyllium husk powder
- 1 tsp baking powder
- ½ tsp salt
- Topping:
- 2 oz. mixed mushrooms, sliced
- 1 tbsp basil pesto
- 2 tbsp olive oil
- Salt and black pepper
- ½ cup coconut cream
- ¾ cup shredded tofu cheese

Directions:

⇒ Preheat the oven to 350 F.

⇒ Combine the flax seed powder with water and allow sitting to thicken for 5 minutes.

⇒ After, whisk in the mayonnaise, almond flour, psyllium husk powder, baking powder, and salt. Allow sitting for 5 minutes.

⇒ Pour the batter into the baking sheet and spread out with a spatula of ½ -inch thickness. Bake in the oven for 10 minutes.

⇒ In a bowl, mix the mushrooms with the pesto, olive oil, salt, and black pepper.

⇒ Remove the crust from the oven and spread the coconut cream on top. Add the mushroom mixture and tofu cheese.

⇒ Bake the pizza further until the cheese has melted, about 5 to 10 minutes.

⇒ Remove when ready, slice, and serve with baby spinach salad.

Nutrition: Calories:208, Total Fat:20g, Saturated Fat:9.1g, Total Carbs:1g, Dietary Fiber:0g, Sugar:1g, Protein:7g, Sodium:446mg

91) Avocado And Herb Spread

Preparation Time: **Cooking Time: 0 Minutes**   **Servings:1 Cup**

Ingredients:

- 1 ripe avocado, peeled and pitted
- 2 tablespoons freshly squeezed lemon juice
- 2 tablespoons chopped fresh parsley
- 1 teaspoon chopped fresh dill
- ½ teaspoon ground coriander
- Sea salt, to taste
- Freshly ground black pepper, to taste

Directions:

⇒ In a blender, pulse the avocado until smoothly puréed.

⇒ Add the lemon juice, parsley, dill, and coriander. Pulse until well blended.

⇒ Season with sea salt and pepper.

⇒ Refrigerate the spread in a sealed container for up to 4 days.

Nutrition: (2 teaspoons)calories: 54 ; fat: 4.8g ; protein: 1.1g ; carbs: 1.9g ; fiber: 2.0g ; sugar: 1.0g ; sodium: 10mg

92) Simple Citrus Vinaigrette Dressing

Preparation Time:

Cooking Time: 0 Minutes

Servings:1

Ingredients:

- Juice of 1 lemon
- 2 tablespoons apple cider vinegar
- 2 tablespoons olive oil
- ½ teaspoon Dijon mustard
- 1 garlic clove, minced

- ¾ teaspoon salt
- 1 teaspoon freshly ground black pepper
- ½ teaspoon dried oregano
- ½ teaspoon dried thyme

Directions:

⇒ Mixer the lemon juice, vinegar, oil, mustard, garlic, salt, pepper, oregano, and thyme in a medium bowl. Serve.

Nutrition: Calories 54 Total Fat: 5g Saturated Fat: 1g Protein: 0g Total Carbohydrates: 1g Fiber: 0g Sugar: 0g Cholesterol: 0mg

93) Cucumber Salad

Preparation Time:

Cooking Time: 0 Minutes

Servings:12

Ingredients:

- 2 cucumbers, chopped
- 2 tomatoes, chopped
- 1 tablespoon olive oil
- 1 yellow onion, chopped
- 1 jalapeno pepper, chopped

- 1 garlic clove, minced
- 1 teaspoon chopped parsley
- 2 tablespoons lime juice
- 2 teaspoons chopped cilantro
- ½ teaspoon dill, dried

Directions:

⇒ In a large salad bowl, mix the cucumbers with the tomatoes, onion, jalapeno, garlic, parsley, lime juice, cilantro, dill and oil.

⇒ Mix well and keep in the fridge for 1 hour before serving as a side salad.

Nutrition: Calories 132Fat 3gFiber 1gCarbs 7gProtein 4g

94) Baked Tomatoes

Preparation Time:

Cooking Time:

Servings:2

Ingredients:

- 2 minced garlic cloves
- 2 tbsps. Olive oil
- 2 sliced large tomatoes

- 2 tbsps. Minced basil
- 1 minced rosemary sprig

Directions:

⇒ Brush a baking sheet with olive oil.

⇒ Arrange the tomato slices on the baking sheet. Sprinkle with garlic, basil and rosemary. Brush with olive oil.

⇒ Bake in a preheated 350°F oven for 5-10 minutes.

Nutrition: Calories: 161, Fat:14.5 g, Carbs:2 g, Protein:0.4 g, Sugars:2 g, Sodium:4 mg

95) Ultimate Roast Potatoes

Preparation Time:

Cooking Time:

Servings:4

Ingredients:

- Pepper
- 2 lbs. baby potatoes
- 3 skinned out garlic clove

- ½ c. stock
- 5 tbsps. Olive oil
- 1 rosemary sprig

Directions:

⇒ Set your pot to Sauté mode and add oil

⇒ Once it is heated up, add in the garlic, rosemary and potatoes

⇒ Lock up the lid and cook on HIGH pressure for 7 minutes

⇒ Once done, wait for 10 minutes and release the pressure naturally

⇒ Sauté the potatoes for 10 minutes and brown them

⇒ Take a sharp knife and cut a small piece in the middle of your potatoes and pour the stock

⇒ Add garlic cloves and peel the potatoes skin

⇒ Sprinkle a bit of pepper and enjoy!

Nutrition: Calories: 42, Fat:1.3 g, Carbs:7.3 g, Protein:0.8 g, Sugars:1.7 g, Sodium:501 mg

96) Green Beans And Okra

Preparation Time: | **Cooking Time: 30 Minutes** | **Servings:4**

Ingredients:

- 1 cup okra, sliced
- 1-pound green beans, trimmed and halved
- A pinch of salt and black pepper
- 3 scallions, chopped

- 2 garlic cloves, minced
- 3 tablespoons olive oil
- 1 tablespoon cilantro, chopped

Directions:

⇒ Spread the green beans and the okra on a baking sheet lined with parchment paper, add the rest of the ingredients, toss and bake at 360 degrees F for 30 minutes.

⇒ Divide the mix between plates and serve as a side dish.

Nutrition: calories 120, fat 1, fiber 1, carbs 8, protein 7

97) Herbed Mango Mix

Preparation Time: | **Cooking Time: 0 Minutes** | **Servings:4**

Ingredients:

- 2 mangos, peeled and chopped
- 2 spring onions, chopped
- 1 avocado, peeled, pitted and cubed
- 1 tablespoon olive oil
- 1 tablespoon chives, chopped

- 1 tablespoon oregano, chopped
- 1 tablespoon basil, chopped
- 2 tablespoons lemon juice
- Salt and black pepper to the taste

Directions:

⇒ In a salad bowl, mix the mangos with the spring onions, the avocado and the other ingredients, toss and serve as a side dish.

Nutrition: calories 200, fat 5, fiber 7, carbs 12, protein 3

98) Devilled Eggs

Preparation Time: **Cooking Time:**   **Servings: 12**

Ingredients:

- 1/3 c. plain fat-free Greek yogurt
- ¼ tsp. ground black pepper
- 1 tsp. yellow mustard
- 1 tsp. white sugar

- 6 large eggs
- ¼ tsp. fine sea salt
- 1 tsp. red wine vinegar

Directions:

⇒ Put the eggs in a large, deep saucepan, and add enough water to completely cover them by ½ an inch.

⇒ Let the water boil, and then cook the eggs for 12 minutes.

⇒ Drain the hot water from the pan and cover the eggs in cold water. Rest the eggs rest for 2 minutes.

⇒ Drain the water and repeat this process until the eggs have completely cooled.

⇒ Peel the shell, and then halve each egg lengthwise.

⇒ Separate the yolks from the whites.

⇒ Use only 5 of the 6 egg yolks, and put them in a small bowl.

⇒ Using a fork, mash the yolks until there are no large lumps, and then add the mustard, Greek yogurt, sugar, vinegar, salt, and pepper to the bowl. Stir this mixture until all the ingredients are well combined and smooth.

⇒ You may transfer this filling to a small plastic food storage bag and snipping off one of the corners of the bag, make a piping bag or you may simply spoon the filling into the egg whites.

⇒ Squeeze the egg yolk filling through hole in the piping bag into the egg whites, and serve garnish with paprika or parsley leaves, if desired.

Nutrition: Calories: 37, Fat:2.1 g, Carbs:0.8 g, Protein:3.8 g, Sugars:0.33 g, Sodium:94 mg

99) Cauliflower Mash

Preparation Time: **Cooking Time: 15 Minutes**   **Servings:4**

Ingredients:

- 1½ cups veggie stock
- 1 cauliflower head, florets separated
- 2 teaspoons olive oil

- A pinch of salt and black pepper
- ½ teaspoon ground turmeric
- 3 chives, chopped

Directions:

⇒ Put the stock and the cauliflower in a pot and bring to a boil over medium heat.

⇒ Cook for 15 minutes, drain, and transfer to a bowl then mash using a potato masher.

⇒ Add the oil, salt, pepper, chives and turmeric.

⇒ Stir really well, divide between plates and serve as a side dish.

Nutrition: Calories 200Fat 4gFiber 6gCarbs 7gProtein 10g

100) Chicken Salsa Soup

Preparation Time: **Cooking Time: 7 Hours**   **Servings:8**

Ingredients:

- 1 lbs. raw chicken breasts
- 2 tbsp. Taco seasoning, homemade
- Oz cubed cream cheese
- 1 tbsp. ancho Chile powder
- 2 tbsp. garlic, minced
- 1 can green chilies and Rote tomatoes

- 1 tbsp. salt
- ½ cup chopped cilantro
- ½ cup chopped onion
- Cups chicken broth
- 10 oz. riced cauliflower, steamed
- 1½ cups shredded Mexican blend cheese

Directions:

⇒ Layer chicken, taco seasoning, cream cheese, ancho chile powder, garlic, Rotel, salt, cilantro, and onion into a slow cooker.

⇒ Pour in chicken broth and cover your slow cooker.

⇒ Cook for about 3-4 hours on high or 6-7 hours on low or until chicken falls apart easily and is tender.

⇒ Remove the chicken and shred it, then mix well the broth with a whisk. Break apart cream cheese pieces.

⇒ Add shredded chicken, cauliflower rice, and shredded cheese. Mix well.

⇒ Use toppings of your choice i.e. Avocado, guacamole, extra cheese, or jalapenos.

⇒ Serve and enjoy.

Nutrition: Calories: 356Fat: 17gCarbs: 6gProtein: 36gSugars: 6gFiber: 2gSodium: 1680mgPotassium: 623mg

101) Stuffed Pepper Soup

Preparation Time: **Cooking Time: 8 Hours 5minutes**   **Servings:8**

Ingredients:

- 1 lb. ground beef
- 2 tbsp. onion, dried and minced
- 1 tbsp. garlic, minced
- Salt and pepper to taste
- 3 cups beef broth
- 24 oz. marinara sauce

- 1 cup rice cauliflower
- 2 cups chopped bell pepper
- ½ tbsp. oregano
- ½ tbsp. basil
- Shredded mozzarella

Directions:

⇒ Sauté the beef, garlic, and onion in a skillet until browned then transfer to a slow cooker.

⇒ Stir in salt and pepper, beef broth, marinara sauce, riced cauliflower, bell pepper, oregano, and basil to the slow cooker.

⇒ Cover the slow cooker and cook for 8 hours.

⇒ Garnish with shredded mozzarella.

⇒ Serve and enjoy.

Nutrition: Calories 193Fat 12gCarbs 9gProtein 13gSugar: 6gFiber: 3gSodium: 826mgPotassium 642g

102) Honey-lime Vinaigrette With Fresh Herbs

Preparation Time: **Cooking Time: 0 Minutes**   **Servings:1**

Ingredients:

- Juice of 4 limes
- 3 tablespoons honey
- 2 tablespoons apple cider vinegar
- 2 tablespoons Dijon mustard

- 2 garlic cloves, minced
- 3 scallions, finely chopped
- ½ cup roughly chopped fresh cilantro

Directions:

⇒ Whisk the lime juice, honey, vinegar, mustard, and garlic in a medium bowl. Put the scallions and cilantro, stir.

⇒ Storage: Store in a screw-top jar in the refrigerator for up to 5 days.

⇒ Substitution tip: For a spicier vinaigrette, add ½ teaspoon of chili powder or red pepper flakes.

Nutrition: Calories 82 Total Fat: 1g Protein: 1g Total Carbohydrates: 21g Fiber: 2g Sugar: 16g Cholesterol: 0mg

103) Rice Pilaf With Almonds

Preparation Time: **Cooking Time: 25 Minutes**   **Servings: 12**

Ingredients:

- 2 bell peppers
- ½ cup almonds
- 3 cups brown rice
- 6 cups chicken stock
- ¼ teaspoon ground white pepper

- 1 teaspoon salt
- 1 cup broccoli
- 2 oz Parmesan cheese
- 1 teaspoon oregano
- 1 teaspoon basil
- 2 red onions

Directions:

⇒ Wash the bell peppers carefully and remove the seeds then chop.

⇒ Peel the onions and dice them.

⇒ Wash the broccoli and separate it into small florets.

⇒ In a mixing bowl, combine the diced onions, chopped sweet peppers, and broccoli florets together. Stir the mixture gently.

⇒ Sprinkle the vegetable mixture with the ground white pepper, salt, oregano, and basil. Stir it well again.

⇒ In a large saucepan, combine the brown rice and chicken stock together.

⇒ Crush the almonds and add them to the brown rice mixture.

⇒ Add the vegetable mixture and stir it carefully.

⇒ Preheat the oven to 350 F and transfer the saucepan with the rice mixture into the oven.

⇒ Cook the dish for 25 minutes.

⇒ When the pilaf is cooked, remove it from the oven and cool slightly.

⇒ Grate the Parmesan cheese and sprinkle the pilaf with the grated cheese.

⇒ Serve the pilaf immediately.

Nutrition: calories: 233, fat: 4g, total carbs: 41.9g, sugars: 2.4g, protein: 11.4g

104) Rice And Beans

Preparation Time: **Cooking Time: 1 Hour**   **Servings: 6**

Ingredients:

- 1 tablespoon olive oil
- 1 yellow onion, chopped
- 2 celery stalks, chopped
- 2 garlic cloves, minced

- 2 cups brown rice
- 1½ cup canned black beans, rinsed and drained
- 4 cups veggie stock
- Salt and black pepper to the taste

Directions:

⇒ Heat up a pan with the olive oil over medium heat, add celery and onion.

⇒ Stir and cook for 8 minutes.

⇒ Add beans and garlic, stir again and sauté them as well for about 5 minutes.

⇒ Add rice, stock, salt and pepper. Stir, cover, cook for 45 minutes, then divide between plates and serve.

Nutrition: Calories 212Fat 3gFiber 2gCarbs 2gProtein 1g

105) Parsley Avocado Mix

Preparation Time: **Cooking Time: 0 Minutes**   **Servings: 4**

Ingredients:

- 1 tablespoon olive oil
- 2 avocados, peeled, pitted and sliced
- 1 tablespoon parsley, chopped

- 1 tablespoon lemon juice
- 1 tablespoon lemon zest, grated
- A pinch of salt and black pepper

Directions:

⇒ In a bowl, combine the avocados with the oil, the parsley and the other ingredients, toss and serve as a side dish.

Nutrition: calories 100, fat 0.5, fiber 1, carbs 5, protein 5

106) Tofu Eggplant Pizza

Preparation Time: **Cooking Time: 36 Minutes**   **Servings:4**

Ingredients:

- 2 eggplants
- 1/3 cup melted butter
- 2 garlic cloves, minced
- 1 red onion
- 12 oz. crumbled tofu
- 7 oz. tomato sauce

- 1 tsp salt
- ½ tsp black pepper
- ½ tsp cinnamon powder
- 1 cup shredded tofu cheese
- ¼ cup chopped fresh oregano

Directions:

⇒ Preheat the oven to 400 F and line a baking sheet with parchment paper.

⇒ Use a sharp knife to slice the eggplant lengthwise of ½-inch thickness. Lay on a plate and brush with some butter.

⇒ Transfer the eggplant slices to the baking sheet and bake in the oven until lightly browned, about 20 minutes.

⇒ Heat the remaining butter in a skillet and sauté the garlic and onion until fragrant and soft, about 3 minutes.

⇒ Stir in the tofu and cook for 3 minutes. Add the tomato sauce and season with salt and black pepper. Simmer for 10 minutes.

⇒ Remove the eggplant from the oven and spread the tofu sauce on top. Sprinkle with the tofu cheese and oregano. Bake further for 10 minutes or until the cheese has melted.

⇒ Serve the dish with collard peppers salad.

Nutrition: Calories:676, Total Fat:63.6g, Saturated Fat:36.5g, Total Carbs:9g, Dietary Fiber:3g, Sugar:1g, Protein:23g, Sodium:1169mg

Chapter 8: Anti-Inflammatory Meal Plan On a Budget

Day 1

23) Delicious Amaranth Porridge | Calories 199

28) Lentil Curry | Calories 290

77) Spinach Cabbage Slaw | Calories 194

41) Pork With Thyme Sweet Potatoes | Calories 210

105) Parsley Avocado Mix | Calories 100

Day 3

14) Perky Paleo Potato & Protein Powder | Calories 302

36) Heartfelt Tuna Melt | Calories 320

88) Frozen Blueberry Yogurt Bites | Calories 91

38) Peach Chicken Treat | Calories 270

90) White Pizza With Mixed Mushrooms | Calories 208

Day 5

7) Buckwheat Cinnamon And Ginger Granola | Calories 220

24) Almond Flour Pancakes With Cream Cheese | Calories 170

79))Passion Fruit Cream | Calories 220

74) Pork With Olives | Calories 280

106) Tofu Eggplant Pizza | Calories 676

Day 7

1) Spicy Shakshuka | Calories 251

37) Lemon Salmon With Kaffir Lime | Calories 103

82) Warm Cinnamon-turmeric Almond Milk | Calories 133

62) Chicken And Sweet Potato Stew | Calories 297

94) Baked Tomatoes | Calories 161

Day 2

26) Cheesy Flax And Hemp Seeds Muffins | Calories 179

32) Broccoli Cauliflower Salad | Calories 259

76) Olives Parsley Spread | Calories 124

54) Pork With Pears And Ginger | Calories 220

100) Chicken Salsa Soup | Calories 356

Day 4

18) Poached Salmon Egg Toast | Calories 389

34) Baked Tomato Hake | Calories 265

87) Cinnamon Pecans | Calories 195

66) Oregano Pork | Calories 300

103) Rice Pilaf With Almonds | Calories 233

Day 6

3) Breakfast Oatmeal | Calories 395

30) Juicy Broccolini With Anchovy Almonds | Calories 350

84) Mango And Nigella Seeds Stew | Calories 140

71) Pork Salad | Calories 225

97) Herbed Mango Mix | Calories 200